Public Health
NURSING
LEADERSHIP

*A Guide to Managing
the Core Functions*

Bobbie Berkowitz, PhD, RN, FAAN
Professor and Chair
Department of Psychosocial and Community Health
University of Washington School of Nursing
Seattle, WA

Jan Dahl, MA, RN
Deputy Director/Lecturer
Turning Point National Program Office
University of Washington School of Public Health and Community Medicine
Seattle, WA

Kay Guirl, MN, RN
Nursing Director
Whatcom County Health Department
Bellingham, WA

Bonnie J. Kostelecky, MS, MPA, RN
Director
Office of Planning and Development
Multnomah County Health Department
Portland, OR

Carol McNeil, BS, RN
Nursing Director/Deputy Director
Island County Health Department
Coupeville, WA

Valda Upenieks, MN, RN
Doctoral Candidate
University of Washington School of Nursing
Seattle, WA

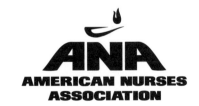

**AMERICAN NURSES
ASSOCIATION**

WASHINGTON, D.C.

Library of Congress Cataloging-in-Publication Data

Public health nursing leadership: a guide to managing the core functions/ Bobbie Berkowitz ... [et al.].

p.cm.
Includes bibliographical references.
ISBN: 1-55810-155-1
1. Public health nursing. 2. Community health nursing. 3. Leadership. I.
Berkowitz, Bobbie, 1950-
RT97 P835 2001
610.73′4′068--dc21
2001022078

Published by

American Nurses Publishing

600 Maryland Avenue, SW

Suite 100 West

Washington, DC 20024-2571

ISBN 1-55810-155-1

PHNL21   2.5M   03/01

Contents

Acknowledgments _____ ix

Introduction _____ x

1 Populations and Performance: Defining the New Public Health _____ 1

Objectives   1

Essential Readings   1

Theme One: Population-Based Practice   2

    Core Functions

    Essential Services

Theme Two: Performance-Based Practice   5

Learning Activities   6

    Learning Activity #1: Ten Essential Services

    Learning Activity #2: Infrastructure Indicators

References   7

Worksheets   8

2 Challenges for Public Health: Trends Affecting Public Health Nursing _____ 15

Objectives   15

Essential Readings   15

Theme One: Changing Financing of Public Health   16

Theme Two: Performance Measurement and Outcomes   17

Theme Three: Partnerships and Collaboration   17

Theme Four: Managed Care   18

Theme Five: Emerging Health Issues   18

Learning Activities   19

    Learning Activity #1: Changes in Financing

    Learning Activity #2: Partnerships and Collaborative Strategies

    Learning Activity #3: Nursing Leadership Skills

References   20

3 Evolution of Public Health Nursing Roles _____ 21

Objectives   21

Essential Readings   21

Theme One: Evolution and Expansion of Public Health Nursing Roles   22

    Case Study One: Changing Roles in an Immunization Program

    Case Study Two: Expanded Roles for Field Nurses

Theme Two: Public Health Nurses are Well Positioned to Assume New Roles   24

Learning Activities   26

    Learning Activity #1: New Roles for Public Health Nurses

    Learning Activity #2: Expanding Nursing Roles

References   27

Worksheets   28

4 Management, Leadership, or Both? _____ 29

Objectives   29

Essential Readings   29

Theme One: Leadership Skills   30

Theme Two: Distinguishing Between Management and Leadership   31

Theme Three: Application of a Management Framework   32

Learning Activities   34

    Learning Activity #1: Distinctions Between Managers and Leaders

    Learning Activity #2: Self Inventory

    Learning Activity #3: Self Evaluation

References   35

Worksheets   36

5 Managing Human Potential _____ 39

Objectives   39

Essential Readings   39

Theme One: Managing Human Potential to Create a Successful Organization   40

Theme Two: Leadership Behaviors for Managing Human Potential   42

Learning Activities   43

    Learning Activity #1: Creating a Vision

    Learning Activity #2: Leadership Competencies and Skills

References   44

Worksheets   45

6 Focus on the Community_____ 49

Objectives   49

Essential Readings   49

Theme One: Community Participation   50

Theme Two: Community Mobilization   51

Theme Three: Commitment to Social Justice   52

Theme Four: The Leadership Challenge   53

Learning Activities   54

    Learning Activity #1: Steps in Community Participation

    Learning Activity #2: Mobilizing Your Community

References   55

7 Managing the Assessment Function _____ 57

Objectives   57

Essential Readings   57

Theme One: Integrated Data Systems   58

Theme Two: Epidemiology   59

Theme Three: Implementing a Community Health Assessment   60

Learning Activity   60

    Learning Activity #1: Indicators for Community Health Assessment

References   62

8 Managing the Policy Function_____ 63

Objectives   63

Essential Readings   63

Theme One: Governance   64

Theme Two: Legal Authority   65

Learning Activities   65

    Learning Activity #1: Comparison of Strategies

    Learning Activity #2: Policy Options Memo

References   69

9 Managing the Assurance Function_____ 71

Objectives   71

Essential Readings   71

Assurance Function Components   71

Theme One: Strategic Development and Action   73

Theme Two: Strategic Management   73

Theme Three: Quality Improvement   74

Learning Activities   74

    Learning Activity #1: Access and Quality Capacity Standards

    Learning Activity #2: Future Scenarios

References   76

Afterword _____**77**

Appendices

    Appendix A. Examples of System Performance Measures _____**79**

    Structure and Policies 79

    Skills and Resources 80

    Information and Communications 81

    Community Involvement 82

    Appendix B. Examples of Health Status Indicators _____**83**

    Appendix C. Core Function Capacity Standards_____**89**

    Health Assessment 89

    Policy Development 90

    Policy Development Capacity Standards 91

    Administration 92

    Prevention 93

    Health Promotion 93

    Health Protection 94

    Access and Quality 96

    Appendix D. Annotated Bibliography _____**99**

    Changing Health Care Environment and Impact on Public Health 99

    Core Functions and Public Health Role Performance 100

    Partnerships and Collaboration 101

    Policy Development 102

    Public Health and Managed Care Systems 102

    Public Health Nursing Leadership 103

    Quality Improvement 104

Acknowledgments

In 1993, a group of nursing leaders from Washington State crafted a document that described how public health nursing could and should practice the core functions of public health. This group of leaders belonged to an organization called the Public Health Nursing Directors of Washington, and the document was titled *Public Health Nursing Within Core Public Health Functions*. Four years later, the same group went to work on a revision of that document. What transpired was much more than an update to the previous document, but a whole new look at how nursing leaders can support the work of population level practice in a public health setting. Now, seven years since the publication of the initial document, this book has emerged, the result of two years of study, dialogue, dreaming, writing, rewriting, and lots of laughter and delight in the company of colleagues and friends.

We acknowledge the guidance and financial support of the Public Health Nursing Directors of Washington. We fondly thank our two research assistants at the University of Washington School of Nursing, Julia Wilson and Laura Land, who spent countless hours reviewing the literature. Special thanks go to our colleagues who reviewed the document and honored us with their critique and valuable suggestions: Nancy Cherry, Chief of Nursing, Public Health, Seattle-King County; Phyllis Schultz, Associate Professor, University of Washington School of Nursing; Sharon Wolvin, Public Health Manager, Tacoma-Pierce County Health Department; Jean Baldwin, Director of Nursing, Jefferson County Health and Human Services; Dorothy McBride, Director of Community Health, Northeast Tri-County Health District; Sandra Owen, Nursing Director, Benton-Franklin Health District; and Shelly Olds, Nursing Supervisor, Lewis County Public Health. A great deal of gratitude goes to one of our authors, Valda Upenieks, who took on the task of editing the document while juggling the demands of her doctoral studies at the University of Washington School of Nursing. Finally, a heartfelt thank you to Elaine Conley, Director of Public Health Nursing, Alameda County Public Health Department, Oakland, California, who has been a longtime friend, colleague, and advisor on this project.

Introduction

Each of us, in our own way, has crafted a style and method of leadership we hope will influence the actions and behavior of the individuals and organizations with whom we work. Ultimately, we hope to influence the health of the communities we serve. However, through some of our own leadership encounters, we have learned that hope, in and of itself, is not an influential and effective leadership approach. Hope can be perceived as the path for our spirit and the dream that urges the heart to beat faster. What is desired in public health nursing leadership, in addition to hope, is the acquisition of new knowledge and the practice of new skills that serve us at a more pragmatic level when seeking solutions, making decisions, and facilitating transformation. Such reasoning led to the development of this book. This guide represents the vision of nursing leaders who have the ideal belief in hope, yet judiciously face the challenge of managing the dynamics of change in the public health arena.

The practice of public health nursing has always reflected the varying social, political, economic, and cultural environments, as well as the changing needs of people. Moreover, the themes that define the core functions and essential services of public health nursing have required the profession to be responsive. For example, in the last twenty years the role of the public health nurse has changed dramatically from the traditional responsibility in communities to more specialized roles, often in clinical settings. Shifts in the future will create further role transitions. The expectations for public health nursing will include performance of community and statewide health assessments, analysis of data and information to diagnose priority health problems and community assets, development of health policy, and assurance that individuals, families, and communities are able to access the health care they need. These activities will require the capacity to track the outcomes of health care, assure the development and evaluation of public health programs and activities, and manage the increasing complexity of finance and governance of today's public health.

As a result of the turbulent and complex demands of the health care environment, public health nursing leadership will demand individuals with a wide range of skills who function collaboratively and effectively. The unique functions and changing features of public health make the world of nursing leadership demanding and stimulating, requiring diverse expertise and knowledge, excellent critical thinking skills, and exceptional interpersonal capabilities. Thus, the field of public health nursing necessitates leaders who adapt to change, are able to take risks, and have a vision for the future. As public health nurses, we hope this book will help you develop and apply a set of leadership skills in managing the performance of the core functions of public health and evaluate the effectiveness of doing so.

We created this book for nurses in public health who have an interest in improving their leadership and management skills and abilities by examining their practice environment, their staff, and themselves. The format offers a thoughtful sampling of concepts, methods, and activities. Chapters begin with objectives that identify the main focus of the topics presented. Following the objectives, themes have been chosen for each chapter that provide a starting point for decision making. Essential reading lists are included next. The content itself addresses the most compelling opportunities and challenges in public health nursing management. Finally, most chapters conclude with learning activities developed to broaden your understanding of the essential material presented. Some activities are composites of different experiences designed to illustrate critical insights. We anticipate that you will find the learning activities challenging and will be able to apply these measures in your everyday practice as a leader in public health.

In the first two chapters, we explore the environment within which public health is practiced. We challenge you to think primarily of the role of nursing with populations and the need to constantly evaluate the impact this changing environment has on the performance of systems. We examine how the performance of the public health system requires specific public health capacity. We also address the public health core functions and ten essential public health services and identify the trends that affect the practice of public health nursing.

Chapters 3, 4, and 5 examine the practice of public health nursing and the practice of nursing leaders. In chapter 3, we describe how new, expanded roles have replaced traditional responsibilities in the domain of public health nursing. In chapter 4, we explore leadership and management skills worth cultivating in order to lead professional nurses who serve populations through assessment, policy development, and assurance activities. Chapter 5 describes how to apply leadership qualities to manage human potential and to create a successful organization.

Chapter 6 focuses on our need to manage strategically while working within coalitions and partnerships to accomplish our goals. We describe the importance of community participation in setting priorities and interventions for public health issues, determine the elements of successful community mobilization, identify the specific skills of public health nurse leaders that support community partnerships, and describe how issues of public health raise ethical concerns for public health nurses.

In the last three chapters, we focus on managing the core functions of public health. Chapter 7 addresses the assessment core function and its required management skills. In this chapter, we discuss data systems, epidemiology, and community health assessments. In chapter 8 we describe the policy development core function. This chapter revolves around the role of the public health governance body and the availability of operating policies and legal authority to manage this core function. Finally, in chapter 9, we review the assurance core function and its specific management skills: administration, prevention, and access/quality.

The appendices include system performance indicators, health status indicators, and core function capacity standards. An annotated bibliography addresses changing health care environment and impact on public health, core functions and public health role performance, partnerships and collaboration, policy development, public health and managed care systems, public health and nursing leadership, and quality improvement.

Enjoy and have fun as you build on your knowledge base about the themes and issues surrounding public health. The expanded role responsibilities of public health nurses make it essential that, as a leader, you can create a positive outlook, project a vision for the future, and inspire a transformation in public health nursing.

Populations and Performance: Defining the New Public Health

Objectives

- Identify two themes that describe the practice and organization of public health nursing.
- Define the public health core functions.
- Describe the ten essential public health services.
- Define two types of indicators used to measure health system performance.

Essential Readings

Association of State and Territorial Directors of Nursing (ASTDN). 2000. *Public Health Nursing: A Partner for Healthy Populations*. Washington, D.C.: American Nurses Publishing.

National Association of County and City Health Officials (NACCHO). 1994. *Blueprint for a Healthy Community: A Guide for Local Health Departments*. Washington, D.C.: NACCHO.

Office of Public Health Practice. 2000. *National Public Health Performance Standards Program*. Atlanta, Ga.: Centers for Disease Control and Prevention. Retrieved October 26, 2000, from the World Wide Web: http://www.phppo.cdc.gov/dphs/nphpsp/index.asp

Washington State Department of Health. 1994, 1996. *The Public Health Improvement Plan*. Olympia: Washington State Department of Health.

As a nurse leader in today's health system, you know how dramatic the changes have been. We have seen changes in the organization of the health care delivery system with a significant increase in the number of managed care entities. We have seen a shift in the traditional mechanisms used for funding public health nursing. The critical health problems affecting populations have changed. For example, HIV/AIDS has shifted from an acute and rapidly terminal disease to a chronic disease. We are experiencing a renewal of the traditional role of public health as we take our place as leaders in prevention and are assuring, but not necessarily providing, access to health services.

We are shifting the focus of public health to the health of populations. Our goal is to promote health, prevent disease and injury, and protect the population from hazards in the environment or biological threats to health. In addition, public demand for accountability has pushed us to clarify roles and to develop and define indicators for improved health and a well-functioning system. As nurse leaders, we are more accountable than ever for measuring and monitoring the performance of our workforce and our public health system.

This first chapter presents two themes that describe the future practice and organization of public health nursing. These unique and interrelated themes are within the domain of influence and management by the twenty-first century nurse leader.

Theme One – Population-Based Practice

This theme characterizes a future practice that focuses on prevention and protection interventions aimed at groups of people. The core functions and essential services of public health are described.

Theme Two – Performance-Based Practice

This theme characterizes the success of future organizations based on how they measure their performance. Systems performance, health status, and risk indicators are discussed.

Theme One: Population-Based Practice

Practice aimed at a population can be defined in part by interventions that shape the overall health profile of a group of people. Usually, the interventions are focused on prevention or protection rather than treatment. Interventions are aimed at the determinants of disease and injury and may be targeted at behavior, such as preventing tobacco use by minors, or at the environment, such as preventing water from being contaminated from toxic chemicals. The understanding of population health has been greatly enhanced through the landmark work of the Institute of Medicine.

In 1988, the Institute of Medicine released a study on the organization of public health and its functions and recommended major transformation (Institute of Medicine 1988). This report started a quiet revolution within public health throughout the United States. In the state of Washington, for example, it was the basis for a series of publications issued by the Washington State Department of Health under the authorship of the Core Functions Task Force (1993), the Public Health Nursing Directors of Washington (1993), and the Environmental Health Directors of Washington State (1993). These papers defined the core functions of public health practice in Washington and described the associated discipline-specific core function activities. In addition, the first *Public Health Improvement Plan* (Washington State Department of Health 1994) was published and became the blueprint for public health in Washington. This report outlined a set of standards specific to the capacity required to carry out the public health core functions. They were defined as assessment, policy development, and assurance. The Department of Health divided the assurance function into administration, prevention, quality, and access. In the *Public Health Improvement Plan*, the core functions were defined in a way that captured the intent of the Institute of Medicine report and evoked a new sense of direction and purpose in public health.

The Association of State and Territorial Directors of Nursing (2000) reference the core public health functions as a part of the analytic thinking process and scientific practice of nursing. They have developed a model that integrates core functions, essential services, and nursing practice. In addition, the new *Scope and Standards of Public Health Nursing Practice* (Quad

Council of Public Health Nursing Organizations 1999) contain standards of care related to carrying out the core functions.

Core Functions

Assessment

Assessment is the regular collection, analysis and sharing of information about health conditions, risks and resources in a community. Assessment activities monitor, analyze and evaluate community health status and risk indicators. During assessment, trends in illness, injury, and death are identified as well as the factors that may cause these events. Environmental risk factors, community concerns, community health resources, and the use of health services are identified. Assessment includes gathering statistical data as well as conducting epidemiological and other investigations.

Policy Development

Public health policy is developed through processes involving many individuals and organizations, including state and local boards of health, elected officials, community groups, public health professionals, health care providers, and private citizens. Public health officials maintain the legal authority to make policy decisions. However, policy is only developed after evaluating information from health assessment activities and listening to the concerns expressed by community members. Public health jurisdictions evaluate both planned and current policies. In order to do this they must have the technical ability and resources to provide authorized decision-makers with periodic information and data analyses regarding specific health issues. A system that facilitates community involvement and informs community members on a regular basis is essential to policy development. State and local public health jurisdictions must have a similar framework for policy development activities while allowing for differences that result from their respective scope of responsibilities.

Assurance

The assurance core function includes activities related to administration, prevention, access to care and quality improvement. Jurisdictions must have a clear administrative structure that supports public health functions. Effective administration is a critical element of all efforts to improve and promote community health. It involves a number of important features, including leadership, planning, finance, and organizational management.

Prevention, health promotion, and health protection activities are at the heart of public health. Health promotion includes health education and the fostering of healthy living conditions and life-styles. Health promotion activities may be directed toward individuals, families, groups, or entire communities. People are assisted in identifying health needs, information and resources, and mobilizing to achieve change. An environment is fostered in which the beliefs, attitudes, and skills represented by individual behavior and the community norms are conducive to good health. Health protection refers to those population-based services and programs that control and reduce the exposure of the population to environmental, personal, and biological hazards that may cause disease, disability, injury, or death. Health protection includes programs such as emergency medical services that are available on a 24 hours basis to respond to public health emergencies. Health protection activities are aimed at the worksite to assure worker safety and at sources of food, water, and airborne diseases.

Quality improvement activities are critical to the assurance core function. Public health jurisdictions participate in monitoring the quality of public health, medical care and social services through credentialing and discipline of health professionals, licensing of facilities, and enforcement of standards and regulations. Efforts to assure access and quality of care require partnerships among many affected parties, sharing of data, and tracking of measurements, programs, and changes over time.

Assuring access to a broad range of health services is central to the assurance core function. With the loss of national momentum toward health reform that would provide basic health care for all Americans, the issue of access is ever present as a major public health challenge. Public health is concerned with addressing barriers to access to primary medical and dental care, public health prevention services, mental health and substance abuse services, and emergency services, among others. Access is one key to reducing the health disparities in our nation (Washington State Department of Health 1994; reprinted with permission).

Essential Services

The core functions of public health are carried out through ten essential services. The essential services can be thought of as a framework within which to place various activities and programs. The essential services, as published in *JAMA* in 1994 (Baker et al. 1994) and adopted by the Public Health Functions Steering Committee in 1995, include:

Monitor health status to identify community health problems: collecting, managing and analyzing health-related data for the purpose of information-based decision making. This essential service encompasses a portion of the activities covered under the assessment core function.

Diagnose and investigate health problems and health hazards in the community: investigating and containing diseases and injuries. This essential service contains activities covered under the assessment core function.

Inform, educate, and empower people about health issues: providing health education to individuals and communities. This essential service contains activities within the assessment, policy development and assurance core functions.

Mobilize community partnerships and action to identify and solve health problems: providing leadership and initiating collaboration. The activities within this essential service are part of the policy development core function.

Develop policies and plans that support individual and community health efforts: This essential service contains activities that are covered in the policy development core function.

Enforce laws and regulations that protect health and ensure safety: maintaining clean and safe air, water, food and facilities. This essential service contains activities covered under the assurance core function.

Link people to needed personal health services and assure the provision of health care when otherwise unavailable: assuring access to services for all vulnerable populations and assuring the development of culturally appropriate care. This essential service covers activities in the core function of assurance.

Assure a competent public health and personal health care workforce: licensing health care providers and facilities, providing continuing education opportunities for the public health workforce. These activities fall within the core function of assurance.

Evaluate effectiveness, accessibility, and quality of personal and population-based health services: monitoring health care providers and the health care system. This essential service contains activities within the assurance core function.

Research for new insights and innovative solutions to health problems: discovering and applying improved health care delivery mechanisms and clinical interventions. This essential service may occur within the assessment, policy development and assurance core functions.

It may seem confusing to have two different frameworks for describing the work of public health. They fit together conceptually, but you may find it easier to choose one or the other. Either way, remember that the language of core functions and essential services is not language that the public understands. It is helpful to describe these functions and services in a way our clients, constituencies, and elected officials can readily relate to. One way to do this is through examples of activities and programs performed within each category. A good reference for this is the National Association of County and City Health Officials document titled *Blueprint For A Healthy Community* (1994).

Theme Two: Performance-Based Practice

Measuring the success of your organization's performance is crucial. The two primary types of indicators relevant to organization and system performance measure the health status outcomes of a population and the capacity of the system to perform. We are skilled at measuring and monitoring the changes in health status of individuals, families, and populations. We may be less skilled at measuring the performance of organizations and systems as they contribute in various ways to health improvement. How do we know which capacities, structures, and interventions are most effective? How do we assure that partners in a health improvement coalition all contribute? No one organization or entity is the sole contributor to health improvement in a population. The interaction among multiple partners brings success; measuring the shared contribution for health improvement is essential. Public health nurse executives must be able to develop these indicators and their corresponding measures for effectiveness. This is a more complex activity than measuring the performance of an individual, such as we do in employee performance evaluations.

Indicators of public health infrastructure measure the capacities and abilities of organizations and systems to carry out the core functions and essential services. In *Healthy People 2010* (US DHHS 2000), seventeen objectives are described that track public health infrastructure. Infrastructure indicators include such elements as the organizational structure and policies of an agency, the skills and competencies of the workforce, the organization's information and communication system, and the processes for assuring community involvement and decision making. For example, within the workforce indicators, one measurement could be evidence that the health department has access to people technically skilled in carrying out assessment activities. For information and communication systems, the health department could show that it has a management information system that tracks financial and service delivery status. Community involvement could be measured by evidence that the health department is identifying and collaborating with constituent groups when addressing the health promotion and protection needs of their community. Other examples of infrastructure indicators can be found in appendix A.

Health status indicators measure the rates of occurrence of specific origins or causes of morbidity and mortality. Health status indicators also measure more global determinants of health, such as social and physical environment, quality of life, well being, and behavior. Health status indicators can be used to measure specific improvements in a population's health. They can also be used to develop a baseline or profile of the health of a community. References to the baseline allow comparisons to be made with regional, statewide, or national data. Our ability to track health status data has been enhanced through the use of Internet-based data sets and geographic information systems that can track and map data to the level of a neighborhood or block. The Institute of Medicine in its book, *Improving Health in the Community: A Role for Performance Monitoring* (1997), offers a model for communities to prioritize community health issues, develop strategies for improvement, and measure their progress toward their health goals. Examples of broad health status and risk indicators appear in appendix B.

Learning Activities

Following are two learning activities to expand your understanding of the essential services described in this chapter.

Learning Activity #1: Ten Essential Services

How would you characterize the programs and activities you manage in terms of the ten essential services? Ask your staff to go through this exercise with you. Use the "Your Health District Essential Services" worksheet to list programs and activities by essential service. An example of how one health department organized their activities by essential service is included ("Northeast Tri County Health District Essential Services").

Learning Activity #2: Infrastructure Indicators

Start an index of the key infrastructure indicators, such as those listed in appendix A, that you would like to measure as evidence of organization and health system performance. Use the "Public Health System Infrastructure Indicators" worksheet provided.

We now turn to a discussion in chapter 2 of the specific challenges that exist in our current public health system.

References

Association of State and Territorial Directors of Nursing (ASTDN). 2000. *Public Health Nursing: A Partner for Healthy Populations.* Washington, D.C.: American Nurses Publishing.

Baker, E., R. Melton, P. Strange, M. Fields, J. Koplan, F. Guerra, and D. Satcher. 1994. Health reform and the health of the public: forging community health partnerships. *JAMA* 272 (16): 1282.

Core Functions Task Force. 1993. *Core Public Health Functions.* Olympia: Washington State Department of Health.

Environmental Health Directors of Washington. 1993. *Core Public Health Functions: Environmental Health.* Olympia: Washington State Department of Health.

Institute of Medicine. 1988. *The Future of Public Health.* Washington, D.C.: National Academy Press.

Institute of Medicine. 1997. *Improving Health in the Community: A Role for Performance Monitoring.* Washington, D.C.: National Academy Press.

National Association of County and City Health Officials (NACCHO). 1994. *Blueprint for a Healthy Community: A Guide for Local Health Departments.* Washington, D.C.: NACCHO.

Public Health Nursing Directors of Washington. 1993. *Public Health Nursing Within Core Public Health Functions.* Olympia: Washington State Department of Health.

Quad Council of Public Health Nursing Organizations. 1999. *Scope and Standards of Public Health Nursing Practice.* Washington, D.C.: American Nurses Publishing.

U. S. Department of Health and Human Services (US DHHS). 2000. *Healthy People 2010: Conference Edition CD ROM.* Washington, D.C.: U. S. Department of Health and Human Services.

Washington State Department of Health. 1994. *Public Health Improvement Plan: A Blueprint for Action.* Olympia: Washington State Department of Health. (Available online at http://www.doh.wa.gov)

Worksheet for Learning Activity #1

Your Health District Essential Services

1. Monitor health status to identify community health problems
   (list programs, activities, services below).

   _____   _____
   _____   _____
   _____   _____
   _____   _____
   _____   _____
   _____   _____
   _____   _____
   _____   _____
   _____   _____
   _____   _____

2. Diagnose and investigate health problems and health hazards in the community
   (list programs below).

   _____   _____
   _____   _____
   _____   _____
   _____   _____
   _____   _____
   _____   _____
   _____   _____
   _____   _____
   _____   _____
   _____   _____

3. Inform, educate, and empower people about health issues (list programs below).

   _____   _____
   _____   _____
   _____   _____
   _____   _____
   _____   _____
   _____   _____
   _____   _____
   _____   _____

4. Mobilize community partnerships to identify and solve health problems.

_____

5. Develop policies and plans that support individual and community health efforts.

_____

6. Enforce laws and regulations that protect health and ensure safety.

_____

7. Link people to needed personal health services and assure the provision of health care when otherwise unavailable.

_____   _____
_____   _____
_____   _____
_____   _____
_____   _____
_____   _____
_____   _____
_____   _____
_____   _____
_____   _____
_____   _____

8. Assure a competent public health and personal health care workforce.

_____   _____
_____   _____
_____   _____
_____   _____
_____   _____
_____   _____
_____   _____
_____   _____
_____   _____
_____   _____

9. Evaluate the effectiveness, accessibility, and quality of personal and population-based health programs and services.

_____   _____
_____   _____
_____   _____
_____   _____
_____   _____
_____   _____
_____   _____
_____   _____
_____   _____
_____   _____

10. Research for new insights and innovative solutions to health problems.

_____   _____
_____   _____
_____   _____
_____   _____
_____   _____
_____   _____
_____   _____
_____   _____
_____   _____
_____   _____
_____   _____
_____   _____
_____   _____

Worksheet for Learning Activity #2

Essential Services for Northeast Tri-County Health District

1. **Conduct timely investigations of community health problems and hazards.**
   - *Communicable disease detection (TB, STD, etc.)*
   - *HIV/AIDS testing and counseling*
   - *Drug labs*
   - *Hazardous substances*
   - *Monitor on-site sewage*
   - *Epidemiology*
   - *Drinking water testing*
   - *Emergency response (spills, flood, etc.)*

2. **Establish systematic process to assess the health status and needs of community and periodically provide this information to the community.**
   - *Assessment – health status, immunization needs*
   - *Birth and death records*
   - *Health status system and information development*
   - *Surveillance (including immunization tracking)*

3. **Mobilize community to set priorities for preventing health problems and resolving health hazards.**
   - *Involvement with community organizations and priority-setting processes*
   - *Provide information on community health problems and hazards to policy makers and the community*

4. **Develop plans and policies that address priority health problems and improve health in the community through a systematic course of action.**
   - *Enact local public health rules and regulations*
   - *Develop an immunization plan*
   - *Board of Health and policy development and action*
   - *Budget development and adoption*

5. **Identify community resources and build public/private partnerships to plan, implement, and manage public health activities.**
   - *Participation in the development of state and federal health policy*
   - *N.E. Rural Health Coalition*
   - *Parenting Coalition*
   - *Breastfeeding Coalition*
   - *County Planning Commissions*
   - *County Solid Waste Committees*
   - *Lake Roosevelt Water Quality Council*
   - *Curlew Lake Owners Association*
   - *Dental Coalition*

6. **Enforce laws and regulations that preserve, promote, and improve the public health.**
   - *Drinking water protection*
   - *Community food protection*
   - *On-site sewage*
   - *Solid and hazardous waste*

– *Vector control*
– *Tobacco sales enforcement checks*
– *Methanphetamine labs*
– *Enforce health codes for schools*
– *Enforce rules of State Board of Health and Department of Health*
– *HIV/AIDS mandatory testing and detection*
– *Communicable disease control*

7. **Implement programs and provide referrals to assure access to personal health services.**
   – *Referrals to area health care and dental providers*
   – *Breast and cervical health outreach*
   – *ABCD Dental Project*
   – *Family resources coordinator (birth to 3)*
   – *Immunizations and vaccine distribution*
   – *Sexually transmitted disease diagnosis and treatment*
   – *Tuberculosis diagnosis, treatment, contact investigation*
   – *Maternity support services and case management*
   – *Children with special health care needs*
   – *WIC*
   – *Family planning*
   – *Referrals of environmental health complaints*
   – *HIV testing, counseling, case management*
   – *Early intervention to prevent child abuse and neglect*

8. **Inform and educate the public on the prevention of health problems and the promotion of changes in knowledge, attitudes, and practices to achieve a healthier community.**
   – *HIV/AIDS prevention services*
   – *Tobacco use prevention*
   – *Sexually transmitted disease prevention education*
   – *Parenting education*
   – *Heart health project*
   – *Food and drinking water safety education*
   – *Nutrition education*

9. **Evaluate the effectiveness, accessibility, and quality of personal and population-based health programs and services.**
   – *Oversight of vaccine delivery and services*
   – *Analysis of client-based data (i.e., WIC, breastfeeding)*
   – *Implement staff development plan*
   – *Analyze accuracy and usefulness of data*
   – *Evaluate effectiveness of public health services*
   – *Staff licensing and certification (nurses, registered sanitarians, health care assistants)*

10. **Develop and maintain efficient and effective administrative services and supports.**
   – *Appoint a health officer and deputy vital records registrar*
   – *Maintain a personnel system*
   – *Maintain a uniform system of financial tracking and reporting*
   – *Establish a fee schedule*
   – *Develop operating policies and procedures*
   – *Maintain a management information system and electronic capacity*

(Reprinted with permission of Tri-County Health District.)

Worksheet for Learning Activity #2

Public Health System

Infrastructure Indicators

List key infrastructure indicators that you would like to measure as evidence of organization and health system performance.

2

Challenges For Public Health: Trends Affecting Public Health Nursing

Objectives

- Identify five trends that affect the practice of public health.
- Identify the competencies public health nursing leaders need to address these trends.

Essential Readings

Association of State and Territorial Directors of Nursing (ASTDN). 2000. *Public Health Nursing: A Partner for Healthy Populations*. Washington, D.C.: American Nurses Publishing.

Courtney, R., E. Ballard, S. Fauver, M. Gariota, and L. Holland. 1996. The partnership model: working with individuals, families, and communities toward a new vision of health. *Public Health Nursing* 13(3): 177-186.

Halverson, P.K., A.D. Kaluzny, G.P. Mays, and T.B. Richards. 1997. Privatizing health services: alternative models and emerging issues for public health and quality management. *Quality Management in Health Care* 5(2): 1-18.

Kang, R. 1995. Building community capacity for health promotion: a challenge for public health nurses. *Public Health Nursing* 12(5): 312-318.

Leong, D., and E. Lewis. 1996. *Health Systems Oversight: A Job For Public Health In The Managed Care Era: Skills Needed By The Public Health Work Force. Report Prepared for the Public Health and Dental Education Branch, Division of Associated, Dental, and Public Health Professions, Bureau of Health Professions*. Washington, D.C.: Health Resources and Services Administration.

In chapter 1, we discussed several themes that describe the practice and organization of public health. Further, we defined public health core functions and listed the ten essential public health services. We also mentioned how in today's rapidly changing public health environment, nursing leadership is faced with critical management decisions based on these core functions and essential services. We recognized that nurse leaders require diverse leadership and management skills to be able to function effectively during these multifaceted transformations.

However, before we explore leadership skills that have been exercised by competent and effective nursing leaders, we must first address the trends that affect the practice of public health. A clear understanding of the environment and issues that influence public health nursing leadership will guide us in effective and innovative decision making.

The themes for this chapter relate to the trends confronted by public health nursing leadership and include the following:

Theme One – Changing Financing of Public Health

This theme relates to reinventing government with accompanying changes in financing for public health activities.

Theme Two – Performance Measurement and Outcomes

Theme two addresses the increasing demands for performance measurement, accountability, evaluation, and outcome measures.

Theme Three – Partnerships and Collaboration

This theme discusses new initiatives that encourage or require partnerships and collaborations among public health, medicine, health plans, and a variety of entities that contribute to overall health.

Theme Four – Managed Care

Theme four examines the influence of managed care as it relates to public health.

Theme Five – Emerging Health Issues

Theme five explores the shift from infectious disease and behavioral risk as the primary causes of morbidity and mortality to new and emerging threats to health.

Theme One: Changing Financing of Public Health

All geographic areas of the nation are responding to a call for lower taxes, fewer regulations, and a decrease in governmental control of the private citizen and individual choice. The public increasingly views government as an inefficient and overly regulated system. This perception, regardless of its accuracy, has fueled changes in federal, state, and local priorities for public health spending. Responsibility and accountability for outcomes are focused locally, yet many local public health jurisdictions are not fully funded to carry out the public health core functions.

In 1995, Vice President Gore initiated a national reformation in government that significantly affected the development of performance measurements, resulting in greater speed and flexibility for action and smaller government size. In part as a result of this national reform, various states and legislatures have regulated the size of government expenditure, placing caps on spending or caps on the percentage of growth in state budgets and taxes. However, the work of government and the public's demand for governmental services have not diminished at the same rate. These demands have forced some state departments of health and local public health jurisdictions to contract and/or privatize some services, thereby downsizing public health.

The challenge for public health nurse leaders, in the face of changing financing, is to develop strategies for new funding sources and mechanisms to support the core functions. Skills to measure results in meaningful ways for varied constituencies will be essential for the public health nurse leader. Emphasis on quality improvement will require nursing leadership to develop an entirely new set of skills in the role of protecting the public's health.

Theme Two: Performance Measurement and Outcomes

Public demand for accountability for health expenditures is increasing. Health departments are being asked to measure their performance and evaluate their programs to justify their budgets. By its nature, public health is less visible than other social and health institutions, is sometimes controversial, and requires long-term interventions to achieve significant outcomes. The general public and policy makers tend to be eager for quick solutions to critical public health problems. Public health departments use community process to address broad determinants of health and function more slowly in developing long-term solutions to social and health issues. We need to look to additional methods, other than the measure of changes in health status, to demonstrate the success of public health interventions.

Public health nurse leaders must look at strategies to support and encourage new methods of evaluation in response to the public's request for accountability. The techniques used by nursing leaders can include measuring performance, benchmarking strategies, and investigating new methodologies for measuring behaviors, attitudes, and other determinants of health. The methods used to gauge success must include both process and outcome measures and evaluate short- and long-terms goals related to public health issues.

Process refers to the sequence or coordination of public health nursing activities. Implicit in its emphasis is the assumption that thoughtful application of the principles and findings of public health nursing will produce excellent outcomes that benefit the community. The comprehensiveness and quality of the process is the key focus for this element of measurement. Outcome measures reflect the net changes that occur as a result of public health interventions.

Theme Three: Partnerships and Collaboration

The new buzz words in health and social service are collaboration and partnering (Lasker 1997; Halverson et al. 1997). Recently, in an effort to achieve improved health outcomes, national groups have established common ground in making broad-based recommendations to schools of public health and medicine, hospitals, and nursing and physician practices to partner and collaborate with other health and community concerns.

Dr. Roz Lasker (1997) collected more than 500 national case studies examining how public health and medicine disciplines collaborate for the improvement of population health. These examples describe teamwork ranging from coordination of clinical individual health services to complex alliances for developing and implementing health system policies and for conducting cross-sectional training and research. The monograph documents the effectiveness of community partnership and collaboration as strategies for process changes in governmental financing of public health, outcome standards, and insurance coverage.

To improve the health of individuals and populations, public nursing leaders must mobilize partnerships with other community organizations to develop methods for facilitation, negotiation, and alignment of competing interests.

Theme Four: Managed Care

Current changes in the health care system have created three different systems concerns for public health: access to care, quality of care, and financing of care. Understanding all three issues is crucial for the survival of public health.

A growing number of states are moving Medicaid clients to prepaid and capitated systems. This transition moves fee-for-service reimbursement dollars from clinical activities provided through public health departments to prepaid and capitated systems. This change in financing creates a more complex system of cost sharing and challenges the ability of the population to access public health services.

Additional issues that arise with the emergence of managed care include concerns over reimbursement for services provided by public health departments to health plan enrollees, eligibility of specific services for certain populations, and the lengthy process for receiving services due to plan approval requirements.

The challenge for public health nurse leaders is to develop methods to facilitate communication with multiple managed care and health maintenance organizations, other payers, and insurance groups. These methods should include establishing negotiations and comprehensive contracts that cover residents of a given public health jurisdiction. It is incumbent upon public health nurse leaders to clearly demonstrate to health insurance providers the strengths and value of public health.

As the provision of clinical services for high-risk populations shifts to managed care, public health has developed a new role in assuring the quality of care. This includes attention to how well managed care contributes to prevention and health protection.

Theme Five: Emerging Health Issues

The causes of death and illness in the United States have changed dramatically. Measles, pneumonia, and influenza had extremely high mortality rates at the turn of the century but have since been controlled through vaccines and antibiotics. Chronic disease currently tops the morbidity and mortality charts and require new types of intervention, causing a great shift for public health nursing. Public health nurses were the experts in providing populations with appropriate and current vaccines to prevent disease. Now, with the shift in the disease paradigm, public health nurses need new expertise, knowledge, and skill levels to effectively address chronic disease.

Social marketing, psychology, and media advocacy have assumed a larger role in the influence of human behavior and thinking. Public health is behind the learning curve in playing a meaningful role in changing and improving community health status indicators that are behavior based rather than caused by a viral or bacterial agent. Consumers have come to expect a magic bullet and quick fix to disease and injury. Prevention is a much harder message to sell to the public.

These five themes bring challenges and opportunities for public health leadership. Public health nursing will be better positioned to operate in a changing environment if new skills and long-range planning are embraced in a timely way. The survivability and quality of practice depend on visionary thinking and strategic planning. Gebbie (2000) used focus groups of key informants to identify the skills and knowledge needed by public health nurses. She has suggested that these skills become course content for public health nursing education and continuing education.

A Metaphor for Public Health

Public health agencies are a lot like fire departments. They teach and practice prevention at the same time that they maintain readiness to take on emergencies. They are most successful and least noticed when their prevention measures work the best.

In another respect, the two are different. Everyone knows what a fire department does; few know what a public health department does. The very existence of health departments is testament to the fact that, when legislators, county commissioners, and other policy makers understand what those departments do, they support them. It is a rare person who, once familiar with the day-to-day activities of a public health department, would want to live in a community without a good one.

(Washington State Department of Health 1994; reprinted with permission)

Learning Activities

Following are three learning activities that address the five themes that affect the practice of public health, as well as the competencies public health nurse leaders will need to manage these diverse trends effectively.

Learning Activity #1: Changes in Financing

Identify any changes in the provision of clinical services in your department that may be due to the loss of fee-for-service revenues. How has your department responded to this change in financing?

Learning Activity #2: Partnerships and Collaborative Strategies

First, identify existing or potential partnerships and collaborative strategies within your domain of practice in public health. Next, identify an access of care issue affecting your scope of service area. Finally, identify partnership strategies that may be able to assist your agency to deal effectively with this challenge. Write out the plan of action, identifying the collaborative efforts. Be creative. This is an opportunity to think "outside the box."

Learning Activity #3: Nursing Leadership Skills

Discuss how the following examples of nursing leadership can be used to address the themes described in this chapter:

— negotiation and monitoring of contracts

— developing indicators to measure performance

— developing new methodologies to measure behaviors

— communicating strengths and values of public health

— community development and mobilization

— strategic planning

— financial management

References

Gebbie, K. 2000. Preparing currently employed public health nurses for changes in the health system. *American Journal of Public Health* 90(5): 716-721.

Halverson, P., G. Mays, A. Kaluzny, and T. Richards. 1997. Not-so-strange bedfellows: models of interaction between managed care plans and public health agencies. *The Milbank Quarterly* 75(1): 113-138.

Lasker, R. 1997. *Medicine and Public Health: The Power of Collaboration.* New York: The New York Academy of Medicine.

Washington State Department of Health. 1994. *Public Health Improvement Plan: A Blueprint for Action.* Olympia: Washington State Department of Health. (Available online at http://www.doh.wa.gov)

3

Evolution Of Public Health Nursing Roles

Objectives

■ Describe the evolution and expansion of public health nursing roles.

■ Describe how public health nurses are well positioned to assume new roles in the changing health system.

Essential Readings

Institute of Medicine. 1988. *The Future of Public Health*. Washington, D.C.: National Academy Press.

Association of Community Health Nursing Educators (ACHNE). 1998. *Graduate Education for Advanced Practice in Community/Public Health Nursing*. Retrieved November 1, 2000, from the World Wide Web: http://www.uncc.edu/achne/chnposition.htm

While the challenges identified in the previous chapters are critical and far reaching, the practice of public health nursing has always reflected the varying social, political, economic, and cultural environments as well as the changing needs of people. This responsiveness has required public health nursing to be an ever changing profession. In the last twenty years alone, public health nursing has evolved from its original role in communities (*i.e.*, assessing community needs, setting priorities, and taking action to improve health) to more specialized, clinical roles. This move resulted from changes in the health care environment, categorical funding for specific health problems, and diminished public health resources. By the mid-1990s, the pendulum started to swing again; public health departments found themselves relinquishing clinical services back to community providers. For the past one hundred years, public health nurses have been responsive to frequent changes in the health system, and as a result, they are well positioned to assume new roles today.

In the previous two chapters, we defined the public health core functions, described the ten essential services, and identified five trends that affect the practice of public health nursing and the organization of public health. In this chapter, we will explore two themes that describe opportunities to move forward and ways of responding to changes in the health care system.

Theme One – Evolution and Expansion of Public Health Nursing Roles

Public health nurses have become skilled in assuring individual and family services. This theme explores expansion of nursing roles, including services to communities and target populations.

Theme Two – Public Health Nurses are Well Positioned to Assume New Roles

This theme offers understanding of how the skills and competencies that nurses have developed with individuals, families, and the community prepare them for new roles in a changing health system.

Theme One: Evolution and Expansion of Public Health Nursing Roles

Across the country, the mission of public health nursing is expanding to encompass new roles. This transformation can be viewed as a continuum of change from individual and family services to expanded responsibilities in the community. The rapidly changing health system, the publication of *The Future of Public Health* (Institute of Medicine 1988) with its emphasis on the core functions of government in the health system, and the delineation of the ten essential services have created additional roles for public health nurses.

Below we have provided examples of how traditional public health nursing roles have evolved over the past twenty years based on the demands of the changing health care environment.

Evolution of Public Health Nursing Roles

Individual nursing practice	→ Member of multidisciplinary team or community coalition
Specialist practice	→ Generalist practice
Nurse as sole expert	→ Collaborative decision making
Implement policy	→ Develop policy
Individual assessment	→ Community assessment
Individual & family-based services	→ Population-based services
Assure delivery of services	→ Assure quality of services
Report output	→ Evaluate outcomes
Academic-based research	→ Practice-based research

We can use two case studies to illustrate how public health nursing roles have responded to governmental demands and community needs. For both case studies, we have provided examples related to the above table concerning the evolution of public health nursing roles.

The first case presentation discusses the public health nurses' role in providing immunizations prior to the late 1980s to mid-1990s and how the role has expanded in today's health care environment. The second case study represents the public health nurses' role concerning firearm safety and how the role transformed from an individual risk assessment to a population risk assessment. After reading the two presentations, you may be able to think about ways in which your own role has changed as a result of the expectations of the current public health environment.

Case Study One: Changing Roles in an Immunization Program

Prior to the late 1980s, most immunizations in Washington State were delivered by local health jurisdictions. In 1989, local health departments began to distribute state-supplied vaccines to private providers without charge for use in their practices. Local health departments were required to account for the number of doses given, age of the child receiving the vaccine, and storage temperature of vaccines in private offices and to assure a re-call system and free vaccinations for those clients unable to pay. By the mid-1990s, local health departments were giving fewer immunizations than private providers, more children were being immunized, and the rate of children aged two who were adequately immunized increased. The role of the public health nurse expanded during this time from direct service with individual clients to a consulting responsibility with private providers. This change includes at least three of the evolving roles: individual-based services to population-based services, delivering direct services to assuring quality of services, and reporting outputs to evaluating outcomes.

Case Study Two: Expanded Roles for Field Nurses

Over the course of several years, a public health nurse observed that firearms were more visible and accessible in the homes she visited. As a result of her concern related to unintentional injuries, she developed a family survey to assess the size and nature of the firearm safety issue. Of the 366 families completing the survey, 45% indicated they had firearms in their homes and 24% of those kept the firearm loaded. Of those surveyed, 26% stored ammunition with the gun and 65% did not use a gun safe or trigger lock. Furthermore, 44% of the gun owners and 73% of their children had not received firearm safety training. The risk of unintentional injury existed not only for these families but for their young friends and relatives as well. After receiving such alarming results, the public health nurse consulted with the local sheriff's department for advice and training of public health nursing staff on how to improve firearm safety in homes with children. A gun safety plan was developed and implemented. As a result of this case review, public health nurses now educate parents about protecting children from gun injury in the home environment and refer families to gun safety classes.

In this case study, the changes include several evolving roles. The public health nursing staff moved from individual-based assessments to a community assessment and added a population-based intervention. Instead of working individually, the nurses developed partnerships with the local sheriff and gun safety classes in a multidisciplinary team approach. Also, the public health nurses moved from sole experts to collaborative decision makers. Finally, in the absence of firearm safety guidelines, the nurses developed a new policy.

Theme Two: Public Health Nurses are Well Positioned to Assume New Roles

Historically and by training, public health nurses are generalists. Their broad education, knowledge base, and skills (*e.g.*, assessment, problem solving, planning, communication, cultural competence, mobilization, and health promotion) allow them to move easily across settings and roles and to adapt to the changing needs of the community (Kang 1995). What makes this set of skills work in the clinical and community setting is critical thinking. The ability to think beyond the bounds of a limited number of options is what makes critical thinking so important for the public health nurse. Bandman and Bandman (1995) have defined critical thinking as the "rational examination of ideas, inferences, assumptions, principles, arguments, conclusions, issues, statements, beliefs, and actions." The ability to assist community members in a decision-making process requires the use of critical thinking, especially as it relates to analyzing options, reporting data accurately, clarifying the beliefs and assumptions held by community members, and evaluating the results of the decisions. Finkleman (2001) points out that the future of health care is not "black or white." Nurses will be required to think critically and strategically to confront new challenges and to be willing to take risks when formulating decisions.

Public health nurses bring to any situation many educational, professional, and experiential assets. Furthermore, public health nurses are flexible members of the health care team, particularly in public, community, and governmental locations. They already possess the theoretical framework and skills for defined government roles in public health. As a result of insight, flexibility, and inclusiveness, public health nurses are well prepared to be at the center of a workforce that will move health departments forward and be accountable in preserving and protecting the health of the public.

Public health nurses can expand their roles in settings that are continuously changing. How and why this occurs can be summarized as follows:

1. *Nurses bring the knowledge of basic human health and illness into the context of public health.* Basic sciences such as pathophysiology, bacteriology, and psychology provide the nurse with knowledge and experience related to the human response to illness, disease, and injury. This knowledge is critical in developing appropriate health promotion and disease prevention interventions (ACHNE 1998; Conley 1995; Salmon 1993). Basic nursing education exposes nurses to the larger health care system and its institutions and places the nurse in a position to create partnerships throughout the health care industry.

2. *Nurses educated at the baccalaureate level bring basic public health theory and population-based practice to health departments.* At a minimum, this education provides introductory knowledge and basic tools in epidemiology, biostatistics, communicable disease, environmental health, policy, and governance in public health. "Public health nurses provide a critical linkage between epidemiological data and clinical understanding of health and illnesses as it is experienced in people's lives" (Wallinder 1997, 79).

3. *Public health nurses bring clinical nursing skills to public health.* Make no mistake, "not all hands-on personal health care services will be taken on by others in the reformed health care system" (Salmon 1993, 1675). In many places, public health nurses will need to continue supplying the excellent clinical care to individuals and families that they have always provided (ASTDN 2000).

4. *Public health nurses move easily across settings, contracting and expanding their roles depending on community need* (Salmon 1993). By being responsive to the changing health needs of the community, public health nursing has developed as its trademark the

capacity and flexibility to shift its focus of practice (ASTDN 2000). Public health nurses are perhaps the most flexible element of a fairly concrete enterprise (Salmon 1993, 1674). They define and redefine their roles as they live them, responding to changes in society, health care systems, and emerging trends (Wallinder 1997).

5. *"As trusted health professionals, public health nurses are frequently able to move in communities in ways not possible for others"* (Salmon 1993, 1675). "For the second year in a row, Gallup's survey on honesty and ethics in professions finds that the American public rates nursing as the field with the highest standards of honesty and ethics" (Carlson 2000). Working closely with individuals and families allows public health nurses to gain the trust of the community. This trust provides the public health nurse with ready access to client populations who are difficult to engage, to agencies, and to health care providers (Conley 1995). Appreciation of the intricacies of community social networks gives public health nurses insight into ways to reach the silent or uninvolved, such as people of color, the elderly, and the homeless. Honest expression of values, beliefs, and intimate concerns is more likely divulged to trusted individuals (Kang 1995). This trust leads to a policy role for public health nurses in bringing needs and concerns of citizens to the attention of policy makers. In addition, they can be "community barometers that provide reality checks" for policy makers (Salmon 1993, 1675).

6. *By virtue of their work in communities, public health nurses are well placed to facilitate the development of coalitions and the mobilization of communities.* Through contact with multiple social groups and agencies, public health nurses have the perfect opportunity to solicit concerns of key members of these groups and organize them into coalitions to respond to concerns in the community. These established relationships allow public health nurses to create alliances with key members of community groups to establish advisory committees, form focus groups, identify primary informants, and develop descriptive methods that are culturally sensitive to individual, family, and community needs, values, language, and cultural differences. Nurses are essential in facilitating community capacity development by encouraging participation, strengthening community health services, and coordinating public policy (Kang 1995).

7. *Public health nurses have immediate knowledge of current and emerging issues through daily contact with high-risk populations.* Public health nurses have health information from individual and family assessments that may not be reflected in traditional statistical data and may be identified before trends in data appear. This early identification of potential health problems in communities provides the opportunity for further assessment, surveillance, and early development of interventions before problems are entrenched. In addition, these individual and family data can be aggregated to the whole population when biostatistical approaches have determined that they are truly representative of the whole. These data on the needs and health concerns of high-risk populations might not otherwise be considered in a community plan (Conley 1995; Quad Council of Public Health Nursing Organizations 1999).

8. *The missions of public health and nursing are similar.* They are both rooted in the promotion of health and prevention of disease, injury, and disability (ASTDN 2000). By combining public health and professional nursing practice, the public health nurse is concerned with all levels of prevention in individuals, families, populations, and whole communities. "A practice focused on prevention is grounded in the eye-witness of life styles and living conditions related to illness and disease" (Kang 1995, 313).

9. The *public health core functions mirror the nursing process.* Nursing is founded in the process of assessing needs, developing interventions, and assuring the interventions are carried out. The public health core functions of assessment, policy development, and assurance include all the elements of the nursing process. "Both are forms of analytical thinking and the scientific process" (ASTDN 2000, 9).

10. *Public health nurses have been the backbone of the public health system for more than one hundred years.* The sheer number and broad distribution of public health nurses throughout the country positions them well for building capacity in communities and filling new and evolving roles (Kang 1995).

11. *Public health nurses can assume leadership positions in the overall management of the public health endeavor.* More generalists with backgrounds in public health sciences, management, and the health professions will be needed to lead public health agencies (Salmon 1993). Public health nurses are already well represented in the leadership of local and state public health agencies, and the need for their skills will continue.

Learning Activities

Two learning activities explore the expansion of public health nursing roles and how nurses are well positioned to assume these new roles in the changing health care system.

Learning Activity #1: New Roles for Public Health Nurses

Based on the changing health care patterns in your community, you can no longer justify keeping your well-child clinic open. Those clients not enrolled in managed care have been referred to other resources, and it has been suggested that you lay off the clinic nurses.

a. What roles might you develop for the well-child clinic nurses in your agency?

b. If you have completed a community assessment, show how it supports these new roles.

c. Develop a rationale for your Board of Health for retaining the well-child clinic nurses.

Refer to the draft set of competencies in the required reading, *Graduate Education for Advanced Practice in Community/Public Health Nursing,* for ideas about new roles.

Learning Activity #2: Expanding Nursing Roles

Identify and give examples of where staff in your agency fit on the continuum of the expanding nursing roles. From your own public health nursing experiences, can you add new categories to the list of nursing roles? Use the worksheet, "Evolution of Public Health Nursing Roles."

References

Association of Community Health Nursing Educators (ACHNE). 1998. *Graduate Education for Advanced Practice in Community/Public Health Nursing.* Retrieved November 1, 2000, from the World Wide Web: http://www.uncc.edu/achne/chnposition.htm

Association of State and Territorial Directors of Nursing (ASTDN). 2000. *Public Health Nursing: A Partner for Healthy Populations.* Washington, D.C.: American Nurses Publishing.

Bandman, E., and G. Bandman. 1995. *Critical Thinking in Nursing,* 2nd ed. Stamford, Conn.: Appleton and Lange.

Carlson, D. 2000. "Nurses Remain At Top Of Honesty And Ethics Poll." Princeton, N.J.: Gallup Poll Organization. Retrieved December 27, 2000, from the World Wide Web: http://www.gallup.com/poll/releases/pr001127.asp

Conley, E. 1995. Public health nursing within core public health functions: "Back to the future." *Journal of Public Health Management and Practice* 1(3): 1-8.

Finkelman, A. 2001. *Managed Care: A Nursing Perspective.* Upper Saddle River, N.J.: Prentice-Hall, Inc.

Institute of Medicine. 1988. *The Future of Public Health.* Washington, D.C.: National Academy Press.

Kang, R. 1995. Building community capacity for health promotion: A challenge for public health nurses. *Public Health Nursing* 12(5): 312-318. (Quotation on p. 25 reprinted by permission of Blackwell Science, Inc.)

Quad Council of Public Health Nursing Organizations. 1999. *Scope and Standards of Public Health Nursing Practice.* Washington, D.C.: American Nurses Publishing.

Salmon, M. 1993. Public health nursing: The opportunity of a century. *American Journal of Public Health* 83(12): 1674-1675.

Wallinder, J. 1997. Supporting one another: The definition of public health nursing, awards, and the impromptu. *Public Health Nursing* 14(2): 77-80.

Worksheet for Learning Activity #2

Evolution of Public Health Nursing Roles

List additional categories of evolving roles.

Current Roles	Expanded Roles

Management, Leadership, or Both?

4

Objectives

- Describe the distinctions between managers and leaders.
- Describe the competing frameworks of public health management.
- Describe how these various roles affect your ability to manage within your organization.

Essential Readings

Kouzes, J.M., and B.Z. Posner. 1995. Leadership Challenge: *How to Get Extraordinary Things Done in Organizations*. San Francisco, Calif.: Jossey-Bass Publishers.

Miesner, T., J. Alexander, A. Blaha, P. Clarkem, C. Cover, G. Felton, S. Fuller, J. Herman, M. Rodes, and H. Sharp. 1997. National delphi study to determine competencies for nursing leadership in public health. *Image: Journal of Nursing Scholarship* 29(1): 47-51.

Stevens, R. 1995. A study of public health nursing directors in state health departments. *Public Health Nursing* 12(6): 432-435.

Wallinder, J. 1997. Supporting one another: The definition of public health nursing, awards, and the impromptu. *Public Health Nursing* 14(2): 77-80.

The very nature of public health is inherently complex. Its unique features make nursing leadership challenging, requiring expertise and knowledge, critical thinking skills, and exceptional interpersonal capabilities. Accordingly, public health leadership demands individuals who can grasp the multifaceted nature of our current health care system and function effectively despite its complexity.

This chapter will explore the leadership and management skills professional nurses need to implement the core functions of assessment, policy development, and assurance. We discuss expertise necessary in changing times, particularly as this millennium will demand public health leaders who thrive on transformation, turbulence, and rapid changes. We will examine three themes that explore this topic.

Theme One – Leadership Skills

This theme reviews leadership skills used by nursing leaders and documented in the literature.

Theme Two – Distinguishing Between Management and Leadership

This theme explains when and how to apply the correct set of skills and provides a framework to develop personal proficiency.

Theme Three – Application of a Management Framework

This theme describes many of the roles a manager may be called upon to perform.

Theme One: Leadership Skills

In these changing and complex times in public health nursing, leaders face challenges to create and reach for a vision of a healthy community and/or environment. This requires strong leadership skills. How do we define strong nursing leadership? Is there a formula for its achievement? If so, we could preface it with "leadership must be a blend of art and science" (Flarey 1996, 9).

Many authors in the field of management in the mid-to-late 1990s describe new ingredients for successful leadership. Particularly relevant for public health nursing are the following:

1. *Envision the Future* (Bennis and Goldsmith 1997; Kouzes and Posner 1995; Stahl 1998): To choose a direction, the leader first must have a "mental picture" of a desirable future path for the community and/or organization. This vision can be as vague as a dream. Yet the vision must be realistic, credible, and attractive to the community. Kouzes and Posner (1995) identify six attributes of vision: future oriented, imaginative, ideal, unique, collective in nature, and representing the future.

2. *Engage in Innovative and Creative Change* (Stahl 1998): Innovation in the workplace must be continuous. The secret to success lies in the leader's ability to give up power and tap into the creative and innovative talents of the people she/he guides. In this way, new ideas emerge, and leaders act as facilitators for redesign and creative change in the work process.

3. *Challenge the Process* (Kouzes and Posner 1995; Stahl 1998): Leadership requires changing the "business as usual" environment. A journey is a good metaphor for discussing what it means to challenge the process or to change status quo. Leaders venture into unknown territory and unfamiliar destinations. They travel from one place to another and step forward to show the direction in which an organization or community is to head. Taking risks is of utmost significance for the leader to create challenges and positive opportunities in the workplace.

4. *Empower Staff* (Flarey 1996; Stahl 1998): The key to empowerment is allowing people to define how they will work in ways that are motivating, stimulating, and fun while achieving the goals, objectives, and mission of the organization or community. To be successful, leaders give up power and explore the creativity of their people. Staff on the front lines are often the best source of innovative ideas.

5. *Celebrate Successes* (Kouzes and Posner 1995; Stahl 1998): Promoting a positive mindset is an important responsibility of the leader. The leader consistently supports people with a belief that they can do what is required. When people believe that something can be done, it is much more likely it will happen. When leaders express confidence in people, they foster success. Success, no matter how small, deserves to be celebrated.

6. *Integrate Ambition with Competence and Integrity* (Bennis and Goldsmith 1997): Competence could be described as doing something right. Integrity is about doing the right thing. Integrating ambition, competence, and integrity can provide the nursing leader the public trust necessary to create significant and lasting change. For ambition to lead to public good, integrity—driven by a commitment to the vision—can lead to the accomplishment of goals and objectives. Furthermore, ambition and integrity must be combined with competence. With ambition, integrity, and the correct tools and skills, a nursing leader can develop a vision and make that vision a reality.

7. *Encourage the Heart* (Kouzes and Posner 1995): Encouragement is serious business. It recognizes each individual's contribution as meaningful. It is about caring for your community, for your staff, for your work, and for yourself. Encouragement is about sharing your passion and creating a supportive, challenging, stimulating environment where everyone is inspired to do their best work.

Successful Leadership Behaviors

1. Envisioning the Future
    - Forward-looking
    - Inspiring
    - Setting goals and articulating a vision

2. Engaging in Innovative and Creative Change
    - Imaginative
    - Enlisting others
    - Creating motivating work environments

3. Challenging the Process
    - Risk taking
    - Courageous
    - Searching for opportunities

4. Empowering Staff
    - Fostering collaboration and team building
    - Supporting
    - Strengthening and influencing others

5. Celebrating Successes
    - Recognizing individual contributions
    - Celebrating accomplishments
    - Planning small wins

6. Ambition/Competence/Integrity
    - Honesty and integrity
    - Determination
    - Competence

7. Encouragement
    - Caring
    - Sharing your passion
    - Inspiring "best work"

(Bennis and Goldsmith 1997; Flarey 1996; Kouzes and Posner 1995; Stahl 1998)

Theme Two: Distinguishing Between Management and Leadership

Why should we distinguish between leadership and management skills? Doesn't it take management skills to be an excellent leader and vice versa? Basically, the answer is yes. However, situations within organizations and communities require the application of different skills: at some times the talent of influencing or creating change, at other moments the ability to create and maintain stability. The key is understanding when and how to apply the correct set of skills to each situation and cultivating this proficiency within your personal leadership toolbox.

Consider these two questions that may, as you reflect on them, make the distinction clear: *do leaders always manage?*, and *do managers always lead?* You can probably think of someone you consider being a leader who does not manage an organization, a group of individuals, or a project. Likewise, you may have experience with managers who do not really "create or influence change" but instead maintain the status quo and are effective at getting the job done.

When we think of *managers,* we think of stability, harmony, maintenance, and constancy. Managers are preservation thinkers. Their goal is to ensure that the status quo runs right, efficiently, and with as few problems as possible. Manager goals focus on the present operations, month-to-month performance measurements, cost and quality, adjusting to whatever comes along, and helping staff to do the same. Thinking outside the box of perspective formulas to develop creative solutions to new events is not within this person's mindset (Kerfoot 1998). Management can be learned by developing the technical skills of financial management and human resource administration.

When we think of *leaders,* we think of times of turbulence, conflict, innovation, and change. Leaders are creative problem solvers who use their imagination to visualize new connections between ordinary events and critically analyze the efficiency of the status quo. They constantly ask the question "what if?" (Kerfoot 1998). Leaders are several months or years out, analyzing scenarios that are about to happen and proactively shaping the present day events in anticipation of the future. Leadership can best be learned by actual life experiences, through successes and failures. The way to learn leadership is to find many opportunities to benefit from a variety of experiences (Kerfoot 1998).

We need leaders, and we need managers. Both are essential to making social systems work. Each position plays a distinctively different role. Within any organization, many tasks and processes must be maintained, improved, and evaluated. These processes do not necessarily require vision to accomplish; they require a very good set of management skills. On the other side of the spectrum, communities need natural leaders who get public ideas on the policy agenda, whether at the local, state, or national level. Many of our greatest nursing "leaders" were not managers but have been effective in instigating change.

Theme Three: Application of a Management Framework

Do you ever feel you are being asked to juggle too many roles in doing your job each day? One minute you must be visionary and innovative, and the next minute you are embroiled in the minutiae of personnel problems. Both are vital to organizational performance, but they require very different skills. This chapter encourages you to examine the roles of management and leadership and cultivate both sets of skills and competencies. For instance, some management roles may feel more comfortable to you than others. They may align closer to your value system and therefore gain preference. Yet your role may require that you lead your staff into an organizational change process.

Quinn, Faerman, Thompson, and McGrath (1996) have described a "competing values framework" that allows the leader to integrate multiple models of management and leadership to ensure choices are available to meet the particular needs of a given situation. The "competing values framework" combines the Human Relations Model, the Open Systems Model, the Internal Process Model, and the Rational Goal Model into a single framework. For more information on each of these models, see *Becoming A Master Manager: A Competency Framework* listed in the reference section at the end of this chapter (Quinn et al. 1996).

The important concept in this management framework is that at any given time, you may be called upon to assume a number of roles. Sometimes these roles compete with each other, but each has its place. The more comfortable you can become in assuming different roles, the more effective a manager and leader you will become.

CHART OF DISTINCTIONS BETWEEN MANAGERS AND LEADERS

Manager	Leader
Administers	Innovates
Maintains	Develops
Accepts Reality	Investigates
Focuses On Structure	Focuses On People
Controls	Trusts
Preserves Short-Range View	Seeks Long-Range Perspective
Asks How And When	Asks What And Why
Bottom Line	Horizon
Imitates	Originates
Accepts The Status Quo	Challenges
Does Things Right	Does The Right Thing

(*Bennis and Goldsmith 1997, 9-10*; reprinted with permission of Perseus Publishing.)

The eight roles include director, producer, monitor, coordinator, facilitator, mentor, innovator, and broker (Quinn, Faerman, Thompson, and McGrath 1996, 15-19):

1. *Director:* The director clarifies expectations through planning, goal setting, problem definition, selection of alternatives, and establishing objectives. The director defines roles and tasks, generates rules, policies, and instructions.

2. *Producer:* The producer will be task oriented and focus on the work at hand. This requires motivation, energy, and drive to accept responsibility and maintain high productivity.

3. *Monitor:* The monitor assures that work teams are performing to specifications, as well as maintains structure and system integrity.

4. *Coordinator:* The coordinator harmonizes the team in a common effort. Once the organization's or community's vision and goals are established, the coordinator then builds on the spirit of pushing forward this common thread and creates a team-building atmosphere.

5. *Facilitator:* The facilitator fosters team spirit, manages interpersonal conflict, and smoothes the progress for forward movement of organizational goals and objectives.

6. *Mentor:* The mentor functions in the role of a wise and trusted teacher or counselor. The mentor provides the strength and answers.

7. *Innovator:* The innovator facilitates change and generates a new image, resources and creative reputation.

8. *Broker:* The broker acts as an agent in negotiating contracts and financial endeavors. This is a political and charismatic role in order to obtain what is needed for the organization and/or community.

You cannot possibly perform all of these roles at once, but you can probably think of times when you have been called upon to assume most, if not all, of them. One of your strategies can be to assure that your staff develops the skills to perform these roles so that the demands of the system can be met.

Learning Activities

Following are several learning activities that explore leadership and management roles in public health nursing.

Learning Activity #1: Distinctions Between Managers and Leaders

Take a minute to complete the form, "Chart of Distinctions Between Managers and Leaders (see page 33)."

*   First, create a list of individuals whom you believe fit into a leadership category.

*   Next, list those persons who fit into the management grouping.

*   Then, list what you consider to be the most distinguishing characteristics of each of those individuals.

*   Now, considering the list of "Successful Leadership Behaviors," (see page 31) return to your list of leaders and managers and add to that list the successful skills that make these individuals effective.

Learning Activity #2: Self Inventory

List your strengths and assets as a leader and as a manager on the worksheet provided. Note in what areas you are competent and where you are less at ease. Indicate how you might add to your skills and competencies in these areas. Record your ideas.

Learning Activity #3: Self Evaluation

Describe a circumstance in which you behaved as a manager, yet the leadership approach would have been more effective, and vice versa.

References

Bennis, W., and J. Goldsmith. 1997. *Learning to Lead*. Reading, Mass.: Addison-Wesley Publishing Co., Inc.

Flarey, D.L. 1996. Reinventing leadership. *Journal of Nursing Administration* 26(10): 9-10.

Kerfoot, K. 1998. Management is taught, leadership is learned. *Nursing Economics* 16(3):144-146.

Kouzes, J.M., and B.Z. Posner. 1995. *The Leadership Challenge: How to Get Extraordinary Things Done in Organizations*. San Francisco, Calif.: Jossey-Bass Publishers.

Quinn R., S. Faerman, M. Thompson, and M. McGrath. 1996. *Becoming a Master Manager: A Competency Framework*. New York: John Wiley and Sons, Inc.

Stahl, D.A. 1998. Leadership in these changing times. *Nursing Management* 29(4): 16-17.

Worksheet for Learning Activity #1

Chart Of Distinctions Between Managers & Leaders

Create a list of individuals you consider to be good managers and/or leaders. Opposite the names, list their most distinguishing characteristics and skills.

Names	Distinguishing Characteristics	Skills

Worksheet for Learning Activity #2

Building Leadership & Management Strengths

List your strengths and assets as a leader and as a manager. Note in what areas you are competent and where you are less at ease. Record your ideas for improving your skills and competencies.

Leadership Strengths & Assets	Skill Development Plan

Management Strengths & Assets	Skill Development Plan

5

Managing Human Potential

Objectives

- Describe four components of a responsive, effective, and successful organization.
- Create a vision statement that incorporates the elements of a successful organization.
- Describe the empowering behaviors of a nurse leader.

Essential Readings

Bennis, W., and J. Goldsmith. 1997. *Learning to Lead.* Reading, Mass.: Addison-Wesley Publishing Co., Inc.

Gunden, E., and S. Crissman. 1992. Leadership skills for empowerment. *Nursing Administration Quarterly* 16(3): 6-10.

Lloyd, P. 1994. Management competencies in health for all new public health settings. *Journal of Health Administration Education* 12(2): 187-207.

Once the nurse leader has inventoried the personal characteristics and skills needed to manage a public health nursing staff and identified areas where additional guidance may be needed, it is time to look at how to put these competencies into practice. In chapter 5, we explore components of successful public health organizations and evaluate strategies to empower staff and the community.

In today's rapidly changing health care environment, every organization must be responsive and efficient in accomplishing the mission and vision of the agency. We want to develop an organization that is proactive and places public health nursing in a leadership position. Two themes in this chapter will address these issues.

Theme One – Managing Human Potential to Create a Successful Organization

This theme describes three essential elements in managing human potential: creating a common vision, empowerment, and assuring a safe learning culture.

This theme investigates specific competencies in four areas for managing your workforce: team building, networking, coordinating, and committee management.

Theme One: Managing Human Potential to Create a Successful Organization

Managing the human potential of any organization is the key to success. An effective leader knows how to support staff in long-term growth and development of their highest potential. Staff will be continuously able to enhance and expand their capabilities.

Bennis and Goldsmith (1997) describe three essential elements of a successful organization: common vision, empowerment, and assuring a safe and learning culture. We believe a fourth component should also be included: valuing diversity. We will explore these four components and relate them to public health nursing leadership. At this point, it might be good to remember that to encourage the heart is perhaps at the foundation of managing human potential (Kouzes and Posner 1995).

1. *Common Vision:* The first component of a successful organization is the alignment of a common vision. A public health nurse leader must articulate a clear, compelling vision for the organization. What does this organization stand for? What does it believe in? Where is it going? Furthermore, everyone in the organization must believe in the vision statement. Not only must it inspire people; it must stretch them as well. It is the guiding light that moves the organization forward (Rosen 1996).

    However, a vision is only as good as its execution. Nurse leaders must always consider what it will take to translate the vision into reality. Thus, the nursing leader must facilitate the creation of a shared vision for a way of working together that supports the mission of the organization. It involves team building and encourages an atmo-sphere and spirit of commitment towards a common goal. In creating this vision, it is important to consider the "quality of the process." The amount of openness and genuine caring the nurse leader possesses determines the quality and power of the results (Senge 1994).

2. *Empowerment:* The second element of a successful organization is empowerment. Empowerment is a process by which people, organizations, and communities gain mastery over their lives. Although the extent to which an individual feels empowered comes from within, relationships with others nurture this process. In public health, empowerment often develops through community partnerships, collaborations, and coalitions. According to Gunden and Crissman (1992, 7), "a feeling of being personally empowered is essential to empowering others."

    When the public health nurse leader decides to implement a philosophy of empowerment within the organization, the transformation can be approached from both an individual and an organizational perspective. First, the staff must acknowledge themselves as being at the center rather than the periphery of the organization. This can be accomplished through joint planning processes and requesting staff to represent the agency in the community. This course of action will establish a decentralized decision-making environment. Second, nurses must be given authority to make decisions for the agency and commit agency resources when they are working in the community. "The person doing the job knows far better than anyone else the best way of doing that job and therefore is the one person best fitted to improve it" (Waterman, 1997). Staff must believe they can make a difference and that their activities have meaning and significance.

Nurse leaders should foster a culture of respect in which staff can actually accomplish things without going through multiple levels of a bureaucratic hierarchy. Some specific ideas identified for relinquishing control include: trusting the process, asking for ideas, widening the boundaries, assisting staff in searching for new opportunities, enlisting others, teaching, coaching and role modeling the way, communicating, goal setting, and being positive (Gunden and Crissman 1992).

3. *Assuring a Safe and Learning Culture:* The third component of the successful organization is a learning culture. A learning culture arises in an organizational setting as a result of empowering leadership and establishing a norm that encourages nurses to develop and implement innovative proposals. In such an atmosphere, staff feel their ideas are respected and also believe their leader values the identification and resolution of structural and operational problems. Nurses need to feel "safe" and take the plunge in problem resolution—safe enough to fail and learn from mistakes, as well as evaluate the process and try again. A learning culture likewise fosters systems thinking. The leader who encourages staff to think about how issues and events interrelate when planning for change cultivates this element.

   The ability of the nurse leader to manage the human potential of a successful organization depends on the extent to which that leader can create a team approach to a shared vision, develop a workforce that believes their contributions are significant, and promote an atmosphere of continuous development and lifelong learning. Recognizing individual achievement, as well as celebrating group accomplishments, provides encouragement throughout the process.

4. *Valuing Diversity:* The fourth component of a successful organization is valuing and recognizing diversity, both in the workforce and in the community. The demographic makeup of the United States population is changing radically in ethnicity. First, as a nurse leader, you must know and understand the changing trends in your community and recognize the values of other cultures and subcultures as they relate to health, health behaviors, and access to health care. This can be accomplished by conducting a community assessment that includes cultural diversity and then planning services and activities to meet the changing cultural needs. In addition, you must train your staff to be culturally competent and to inspire trust and confidence among the culturally diverse people in your community (Huber 2000).

   Second, as a nursing leader, you must take positive steps to encourage increased participation of persons from other cultures in the nursing profession (Huber 2000). When possible, staffing in the agency should mirror local demographics. When this is not possible, the nursing leader should consider an outreach program into minority communities to recruit high school and college students into the nursing profession.

   Recruiting, hiring, and training persons from other cultures must be a priority.

   Third, nursing leaders can foster understanding and acceptance in the work environment by organizing culturally diverse teams. In addition, appreciation for cultural differences can be increased by recognizing and acknowledging the unique cultural contributions from the varied heritage of all your staff. Irish traditions differ from Italian traditions, which differ from African traditions and so on. All affect the work environment and create a rich tapestry from which to reach out and connect with community members to develop programs to improve health.

Rowland and Rowland (1997) provide guidelines for nurse leaders who are working to improve cultural diversity in their agencies. These guidelines include encouraging leaders and staff to discuss diversity issues openly, mediating between the personal and professional needs of employees, providing diverse groups of employees the opportunity to solve problems together, and assuring that the organization's culture, norms, and values are explained to all workers.

Cultural competence and cultural diversity have been emerging issues in the health arena for a number of years. Public health nursing leaders are in a position to integrate community values in the workplace, develop a culturally competent workforce, and advocate for the changing needs of changing communities.

Four Elements for a Successful Organization

1. Common Vision
- Develop a unique picture of the future
- Focus collective energy
- Build a commitment to take personal responsibility

2. Empowerment
- Put staff at the center of the organization
- Always say "we"
- Share critical decision making
- Create a culture of respect
- Listen to your staff

3. Assuring a Learning Culture
- Encourage innovation
- Learn from mistakes
- Develop competence: yours and others
- Foster systems thinking
- Encourage your staff to listen to each other

4. Valuing Diversity
- Know your community
- Integrate diversity in the workplace
- Be a cultural ambassador

(Bennis and Goldsmith 1994, Gibson 1991, Gunden and Crissman 1992, Rosen 1996, Senge 1994.)

Theme Two: Leadership Behaviors for Managing Human Potential

In addition to discussing four components of a responsive and successful organization, we thought it would be helpful at this point to elaborate on the leadership and management behaviors described in chapter 4. Peter Lloyd (1994) divided people management into four main categories: team building, networking, coordinating, and committee management. The following list is taken from Lloyd's "catalog of competencies." You may want to identify areas of your strengths and weaknesses in leading and managing organizations as you read through this list in managing human potential (Lloyd 1994).

1. Team Building

- Developing personal relationships by building trust, breaking down barriers with other professionals, and being sensitive to others.

- Letting staff be flexible.

- Having the confidence to delegate.

- Knowing strengths and weaknesses, cultivating the strengths, and giving support through the weaknesses.

- Consensus building.

- Knowing what to delegate and to whom, and how to "let go."

- Fostering cohesion.

- Resolving conflict, mediating, and motivating.

2. Networking

   • Network building and fostering networking in others within the public health sector, across departments and in the community.

   • Attracting the right people.

3. Coordinating

   • Coordinating activities (as opposed to perpetuating hierarchical structures) by integrating and blending team members with a wide variety of skills, backgrounds, and/or locations into a single functioning unit.

   • Exhibiting cooperation and obtaining it from others.

4. Committee Management

   • Getting constituency groups together.

   • Managing committees through presentation skills, coalition building, persuasion, and consultation.

Learning Activities

The following learning activities provide excellent examples of how to inspire, encourage, and nurture a workforce.

Learning Activity #1: Creating a Vision

An important component of a successful and productive workforce is the alignment of a common vision. If your organization has a vision statement, identify how the statement integrates that concept. How was it created? By whom? Do the words reflect an organization "buy-in"? Use the worksheet entitled, "Vision Statement," to record your observations.

If your agency has not formulated its own vision statement, read through the two examples provided. Then, with your staff, create a vision statement for your organization or analyze the examples provided.

Learning Activity #2: Leadership Competencies and Skills

Read the two articles as Essential Reading for this chapter. After reviewing the articles, evaluate your strengths and weaknesses in managing the human potential in your organization. Use the worksheet entitled, "Managing Human Potential."

References

Bennis, W., and J. Goldsmith. 1997. *Learning to Lead*. Reading, Mass.: Addison-Wesley Publishing Co., Inc.

Gison, C.H. 1991. A concept analysis of empowerment. *Journal of Nursing Administration* 16: 354-361.

Gunden, E., and S. Crissman. 1992. Leadership skills for empowerment. *Nursing Administration Quarterly* 16(3): 6-10.

Huber, D. 2000. *Leadership and Nursing Care Management*, 2nd ed. Philadelphia, Pa.: W.B. Saunders Company.

Kouzes, J.M., and B.Z. Posner. 1995. *The Leadership Challenge: How to Get Extraordinary Things Done in Organizations*. San Francisco, Calif.: Jossey-Bass Publishers.

Lloyd, P. 1994. Management competencies in health for all new public health settings. *Journal of Health Administration Education* 12(2): 205-206.

Rowland, H., and B. Rowland. 1997. *Nursing Administration Handbook*. Gaithersburg, Md.: Aspen, Inc.

Rosen, R.H. 1996. *Leading People: Transforming Business From the Inside Out*. New York: Penguin Books.

Senge, P. 1994. *The Fifth Discipline Fieldbook: Tools, Techniques & Reflections for Building a Learning Organization*. New York: Doubleday.

Waterman, R.H., Jr. 1997. *The Renewal Factor*. New York: Bantam Books.

Worksheet for Learning Activity #1

Vision Statement

Identify how your Vision Statement (or the examples of Vision Statements on the following pages) integrates the element of a successful organization described as the "alignment of a common vision."

Vision Statement Example

Southwest Washington Health District

We are seen by the community as an advocate and leader in its collective efforts to become a healthy community with the highest quality of life. We contribute significantly to improving the health of the community through effective performance of our core functions of assessment, policy development, prevention, assurance, and administration. We respond to the community's changing needs, always open to new ways of protecting and promoting health.

Partnerships

We work closely with community members, groups, and organizations, sharing information, finding common ground, and collaborating on mutual priorities while respecting community preferences and values.

Assessment and Policy Development

We help gather, analyze, and interpret information describing the community. Together, we use the information to develop policies and address priority health needs.

Assuring Access

We are effective in our efforts to see that all residents of the community receive health services when they need them.

Prevention Through Education and Community Empowerment

We help the community increase its knowledge to improve health, safety, and environment. We strive to inspire a sense of personal commitment as a strategy to achieve high level wellness.

Environmental Stewardship

We work for high standards of environmental livability, including protection of our soil, water, air, and food supply and model responsible stewardship of our land and natural resources, leaving it healthier for the next generation.

Work Place Culture

Our staff are creative, committed, and compassionate in their work. Encompassing all disciplines, they work together to achieve Health District goals. The organization honors diversity and supports employee learning, growth, and initiative.

Excellence

We are committed to excellence in our work, and we advocate for quality from all health care providers serving the community.

(Reprinted by permission of Southwest Washington Health District.)

Mission Statement Example

Thurston County

Board of County Commissioners

- The Thurston County Mission is to provide quality, timely, and responsive service to the residents of Thurston County in the most cost-effective manner.

- The Mission of the Thurston County Public Health Department is to protect and promote the health of the Thurston County Community, now and in the future.

Vision Statement

- Our Department makes a positive, material difference in the health and well being of the people of Thurston County.

- We achieve our mission . . .

Core Values

1. We see the Health Department as an integral part of the greater Thurston County Community and actively seek cooperation with and input from individuals, jurisdictions, and other organizations to meet the health needs of the community.

2. We value the knowledge, skills, and expertise of all departmental employees; we seek input and contribution to policy development and the shaping of high quality service delivery; we value the strength of teamwork and the flexibility and cooperation necessary to make teams work effectively.

3. We are responsive to and show respect to members of the public, to individuals in other organizations, and to fellow employees. We encourage diversity of perspective while honoring adopted decision-making processes and authority.

4. We value sound data and reliable information on which to base decisions and choices. We work to understand community change and are responsive to changing needs.

5. We value and expect responsible use of the resources entrusted to the department.

6. We prioritize methods to achieve public health that inform, advise, direct, and, lastly, control.

7. We understand and value the need for a long-term perspective. We can and do make efforts, which will bear fruit years or decades from the time of effort.

(Reprinted by permission of the Thurston County Public Health Department; statement developed jointly by employees of the department.)

Worksheet for Learning Activity #2

Managing Human Potential

Competencies and Skills

Strengths	Areas For Improvement

6

Focus on the Community

Objectives

■ Describe the importance of community participation in setting priorities and interventions for public health issues.

■ Determine the elements of successful community mobilization.

■ Identify specific skills of public health nurses and nursing leaders that support community partnerships.

■ Describe how issues of public health importance raise ethical concerns for public health nurses.

Essential Readings

Kang, R. 1995. Building community capacity for health promotion: A challenge for public health nurses. *Public Health Nursing* 12(5): 312-318.

Kretzman, J., and J. McKnight. 1993. *Building Communities From the Inside Out; A Path Toward Finding and Mobilizing a Community's Assets.* Evanston, Ill.: Institute for Policy Research.

Krieger, N. 1990. On becoming a public health professional: reflections on democracy, leadership, and accountability. *Journal of Public Health Policy* 11(4): 412-418.

In the last two chapters, we described leadership and management skills public health nurse leaders will want to develop. Now we will broaden our focus to the community level. In the rapidly changing health environment, public health nursing leaders must frame the transition of public health from its emphasis on providing clinical services to the most disadvantaged individuals to a broader mission of providing essential services to the entire community. *This transition will require a change in the way public health nurses and leaders view their mission and role.* To facilitate this shift, public health nurse leaders must give up control over the agenda and direction of public health interactions and encourage community participation in identifying issues affecting the lives of citizens. In addition, they must develop and implement plans for change and build community strength, self-sufficiency, and well being.

In this chapter, we will discuss how public health nursing leadership skills lend themselves to building the capacity of communities to address public health issues. We will focus on four themes.

Theme One – Community Participation

This theme describes how the development of partnerships and community participation is essential for building community capacity in planning and implementing programs.

Theme Two – Community Mobilization

This theme describes how community building leads to empowerment and challenges public health leaders to think in new ways.

Theme Three – Commitment to Social Justice

This theme discusses how nursing leaders can address health disparities at the community level.

Theme Four – The Leadership Challenge

This theme describes how changing our attitudes and organizational structures can contribute to the development of community capacity for mobilization and action.

Theme One: Community Participation

The development of community capacity through active coalition and partnership development builds from the principle that the community is at the center of this process, and participation by community members is of high value. What constitutes community participation? Minkler and Wallerstein (1997) have proposed that community participation means a sharing of power and responsibility. The movement of community members toward active participation in community development may be elicited through a series of relationships (partnership building) and through what Wolff and Kaye (1995) call "The Six Rs of Participation." Kaye states that people need to be *recognized* for their service to their community and organizations. They need to be *respected* by their peers for the work they do. Individuals need to be given a specific *role*. *Relationships* can be important to people seeking mutual support and friendship. People generally want to be *rewarded* in some way for joining an activity, and the reward must outweigh the costs of membership. And, finally, the *results* of the activity can help attract new members and maintain current members.

The Six "Rs" of Participation
1. Recognition
2. Respect
3. Role
4. Relationship
5. Reward
6. Results
(Wolfe and Kaye 1997)

Public health nurses can be an important link between individuals and the extent to which they develop a sense of participation. They are also essential to identifying community capacity and responding to issues of public health concern. Their strength comes from their familiarity with the internal working of communities and the lives of people in them (Kang 1995).

By working with multiple social groups and agencies, public health nurses have the perfect opportunity to solicit the concerns of key citizens and facilitate the development of partnerships to respond to common issues in the community. Past methods of interaction included networking, coordination, and cooperation. These interactions have been rooted in the exchange of information, altering activities for mutual benefit, sharing resources, or enhancing capacity to achieve a common purpose. Public health nurse leaders advocate for the need to listen to the community and then assure that their needs are heard.

In this new environment, the development of partnerships is vital for building community capacity to participate in planning, organizing, and implementing health programs. A partnership implies equality in levels of status, control, and responsibility among the participants and is built on mutual respect, trust, and confidence. Also, collaboration requires that participants have the integrity to uphold agreements and the willingness to work together to achieve shared goals. Partnerships provide an opportunity to stimulate community members to think about the political, social, and cultural context of health and shape the assessment of community concerns, policy development related to culturally appropriate interventions, and assurance of essential services.

Public health nurses have had substantial success in engaging communities. They may work with community groups to propose new programs and changes in policies. They may also encourage communities to participate in developing research to examine the effect of health policies on a variety of issues, such as access to services, efficacy of programs, adequacy of fiscal allocation, community participation, organizational linkages, and health status of community residents. Through knowledge of community concerns from research and informal sources, communities and public health nurses can lobby for changes in health policy at public forums, legislative hearings, and city/county council meetings. The community's contribution to health needs assessments and public policy activities creates ownership in assuring public health programs and accountability for outcomes.

Theme Two: Community Mobilization

Community mobilization is a process by which community groups identify common goals and mobilize assets to implement strategies that address local concerns. This collective response stimulates and channels public interests, energies, and resources to bring about changes or improvements in the health of a community. The design and implementation of community mobilization is a partnership in which participants work with health professionals to gain understanding of personal, social, economic, and political forces to take control of their lives and improve their life situations. Implicit in this process is the concept of empowerment. Empowered community groups can provide advice on policy development, processes for building systems, strategies to overcome gaps in knowledge, opportunities to bring the community into local planning, and methods to change attitudes.

Paradigm Shift in Community Mobilization

OLD	NEW
Focus on deficits	Focus on assets
Problem response	Opportunity identification
Emphasis on agencies	Emphasis on associations, business, agencies, churches
Focus on individuals	Focus on community
See individuals as clients	See individuals as citizens
Treat individual problems	Develop individual potential

(Adapted from Kretzman and McKnight 1993)

Another area of challenge relates to the values and beliefs of individual public health nurses. Traditionally the role of the nurse has been to provide answers to health concerns and questions in a nurse-client interaction. As students, many nurses were given little opportunity to develop the skills necessary to practice effectively in a community setting. Moving from the role of health expert to community partner can be difficult. Listening and valuing the agenda of others in a community setting can be unfamiliar and uncomfortable territory. This may lead to resistance and a lack of commitment or support for a community process. As a public health nurse leader, it will be your responsibility to coach your staff to see the big picture of health, to participate as a community team member, and to value the beliefs of others as valid perceptions. Ultimately, public health nurses must trust that community process is an essential component of improving health outcomes.

Theme Three: Commitment to Social Justice

In our society, fundamental differences remain as to whether health is a right or a privilege. A survey conducted by the *Washington Post* asked individuals their opinion on the health issues of the 2000 presidential election (Conversation with Robert Blandon 2000). Respondents said:

1. The health system is not working.

2. The government should guarantee universal health coverage.

3. The government is too powerful.

4. The government will not solve the health care issue correctly.

5. The government should go no further in paying for health care.

The conflicts between statements 1 and 2 and 3 through 5 are reflected in national health policy decisions. Inequity in access to comprehensive health care continues to grow amid economic growth (Mechanic 2000). Significant segments of the population suffer from diseases related to poverty and chronic conditions that, left untreated, lead to premature death and disability. Disproportionately large numbers of women and children are uninsured, poorly nourished, jobless, homeless, and victims of domestic and community violence.

A central ethical issue in the health of communities relates to remediation of inequities in the distribution of resources. The nursing leader must be an advocate for affordable, accessible health care for all. To achieve a healthy community, the health issues of all members of the community must be addressed.

The ethical framework of public health nursing practice uses advocacy to address the problems of distribution and access to essential services as well as the cost and financing of health care. If we are serious about eliminating health disparities in our society, public health nursing leaders must speak out about injustice and be prepared to take up the fight within the nursing profession, with individuals, and in the broader society. Nurses are well positioned to work on problems of distribution of health and related services such as housing, protection from violence, nutrition, and public assistance programs. Ways public health nurses can be helpful include the following (Chafey 1996):

1. Identifying Issues

   • Identifying community groups such as the elderly, youth, and minority groups and involving them in planning and problem solving.

- Participating in partnerships with special interest groups and coalitions in the community in identifying issues such as clean air, water, soil and food, emergency services, occupational hazards, providing shelter for the homeless, assisting elderly, nutritional services, violence, and increasing awareness of the effects of racism.

2. Informing the Community

   - Being a spokesperson and advocate.

   - Bringing to the attention of local, county and state level policy makers the need for essential services by those either locked out or invisible to the system.

   - Advocating or negotiating with policy makers for needed resources on behalf of groups that are unable to negotiate for themselves.

3. Empowering

   - Helping both elected officials and the electorate understand and value the public health agenda.

   - Working through community organizations and local government and voluntary agencies to empower communities to address distribution problems.

   - Activating communities to be concerned about problems affecting the community as a whole.

(Reproduced by permission of the National League for Nursing.)

Theme Four: The Leadership Challenge

The leadership functions related to building community participation, community mobilization, and striving for social justice require very specific skills. Communities that define their own problems, control their own programs, and develop their own strategies for change are more likely to have successful, sustainable programs. Public health nurses can act as a resource, consultant, facilitator, educator, advocate, and role model. Public health nurses can take the public health message to the community. They can advise on policies, build systems, overcome gaps in knowledge, forge common understanding and trust, reduce isolation felt by citizens and staff, bring community into local planning, and change attitudes. For public health nurses to be successful in working with coalitions, they must believe in and value the process of community development and empowerment and be able to relinquish control. They must have expertise in facilitating group process, problem solving, building community capacity, social action, and social change. Public health nurses must have a broad concept of health and the antecedents of health, be willing to function as community educators, and respect the diversity of community members.

Public health nurse leaders can help their staff to identify partnerships that will be mutually beneficial and encourage linkages with outside resources. To build a foundation for partnerships, they must build productive relationships with mutual understanding of constraints, requirements, and philosophies. The leader will need to help staff understand that a good working relationship is one that can deal constructively with differences and balance emotion with reason, understanding, and acceptance.

A major issue influencing the ability of nurses to practice within a community development role relates to the structure and policies of organizations in which they practice. Issues of power and authority within organizations will also affect the development and maintenance of a community development role for nurses. Public health nursing leaders must assure the organization is willing to share power with the community and support the community development role by formulating well-articulated policies and allocating adequate resources for the work. Because community development work is not as well delineated or quantifiable as other components of public health nursing, managers must develop standards for evaluating nurses' performance to avoid public health nursing role conflict, role overload, and burnout (Chalmers and Bramadat 1996).

In summary, the time to fully engage communities to participate in public health policy development is at hand. Without citizen support, nurse leaders will find a difficult environment in which to practice. Without constituency backing, funding will erode, programs will not achieve their goals, and public health will fail in its overarching mission of "assuring conditions in which people can be healthy" (Institute of Medicine 1988). This mission cannot be fulfilled unless nurse leaders challenge their organizations and staff to put the "public" back into public health.

Learning Activities

Following are two learning activities that address the development of community participation and the establishment of a community mobilization action plan.

Learning Activity #1: Steps in Community Participation

Think about your current role as a leader. How would you increase community participation to solicit concerns and develop partnerships to respond to current public health issues? Use the format outlined—the six "Rs" of participation—on page 50 as a guide in outlining your plan to stimulate participation and community success.

Learning Activity #2: Mobilizing Your Community

As a public health nurse leader, you have been requested to identify a health care issue affecting the local community that you serve and to develop an action plan to address this concern. Your focus is community mobilization and partnership.

a. How would you go about developing this action plan?

b. How would you identify an issue to address?

Use the figure, *Paradigm Shift in Community Mobilization,* on page 51 as a guide in developing your plan.

References

Chafey, K. 1996. Ethical paradigms for community-based care. *Perspectives on Community* 17(1): 11-15.

Chalmers, K.I., and I.J. Bramadat. 1996. Community development: theoretical and practical issues for community health nursing in Canada. *Journal of Advanced Nursing* 24: 719-726.

A conversation with Robert Blandon about public opinion and health care, nursing, and the 2000 presidential election. 2000. *Nursing Outlook* 48: 203-210.

Institute of Medicine. 1988. *The Future of Public Health*. Washington, D.C.: National Academy Press.

Kang, R. 1995. Building community capacity for health promotion: a challenge for public health nurses. *Public Health Nursing* 12(5): 312-318.

Kretzman, J., and J. McKnight. 1993. *Building Communities From the Inside Out*. Evanston, Ill.: Institute for Policy Research.

Mechanic, D. 2000. Rediscovering the social determinants of health. *Health Affairs* 19(3): 269-276.

Minkler, M., and N. Wallerstein. 1997. Improving health through community organization and community building. In *Community organizing and community building for health*, edited by Meredith Minkler. New Brunswick, N.J.: Rutgers University Press.

Wolff, T., and G. Kaye. 1995. *From the Ground Up: A Workbook on Coalition Building and Community Development*. Amherst, Mass.: AHEC/Community Partners: 100-102.

7

Managing the Assessment Function

Objectives

- Describe the assessment core function.
- Identify the specific management skills required for the assessment function.
- Develop a work plan for performing a community assessment.
- Develop a set of indicators you could use to evaluate your agency's performance of a community assessment.

Essential Readings

Washington State Department of Health. 1996. *Public Health Improvement Plan: A Blueprint for Action.* Olympia: Washington State Department of Health.

Mendelson, D., and E. Salinsky. 1997. Health information systems and the role of state government. *Health Affairs* 16(3): 106-119.

Quad Council of Public Health Nursing Organizations. 1999. *Scope and Standards of Public Health Nursing Practice.* Washington, D.C.: American Nurses Publishing.

Let's review the assessment core function. Health assessment means the regular collection, analysis, and sharing of information about health conditions and resources in a community. Assessment activities monitor, analyze, and evaluate community health status, risk indicators, and, when necessary, health emergencies. They identify trends in illness, injury, and death and the factors that may cause these events. Evaluation measures also identify environmental risk factors, community concerns, community health resources, and the use of health services. Assessment includes gathering statistical data as well as conducting epidemiological and other investigations (Washington State Department of Health, 1996).

Assessment is a broad systematic process for examining current status of conditions in your community. In gathering information on the level of risk and root causes of priority health issues in your community, you may want to adopt a model for assessment such as APEXPH,

PATCH, or CHART, or perhaps you will develop a model of your own (NACCHO 2000, CDC 1995, Missouri Department of Health 1996).

Three themes guide the development of skills essential to managing the assessment core function.

Theme One – Integrated Data Systems

Without access to an integrated data network, it is difficult, if not impossible, for staff to collect health status data. Your job as a leader is to assure access to a network or facilitate the development of the network.

Theme Two – Epidemiology

Epidemiology is one of the most important aspects to the assessment core function. Your responsibility as a manager is to the set policies based on data derived from an information system grounded in epidemiology.

Theme Three – Implementing a Community Health Assessment

In implementing the steps of a community health assessment, you may be called upon to exercise a variety of skills.

Theme One: Integrated Data Systems

As stated in the Washington State *Public Health Improvement Plan* (1996), "Accurate, relevant, and timely information is essential to guide public health policies and for evaluating the effectiveness of those policies." Information collection is the first phase of conducting a health assessment. Data must be identified and assembled to determine how prevalent risks are in a particular community. You must identify what is available, determine what additional data are needed, and develop a plan to collect it. Data collection, storage, and analysis are traditional functions of public health. In the current health care environment, however, data are collected and analyzed in many sectors of the health system and other community entities. Much of the needed information is not available in a public health database. For instance, data from purchasers of health care and health plans may not be available to public health managers. To make decisions on what programs and activities to develop and where to target interventions, public health managers must have access to all pertinent information. Yet how does a manager gain access to information outside the traditional public health database?

An integrated data system combines data from public and private providers through electronic methods so that access to and standardization of data are possible. Data confidentiality is of highest priority, as is the ability to compare data across communities and systems. Creating an integrated data system in which many members of the community participate is one of our challenges in public health. (See appendix B for examples of data sets on injury and violence obtained outside the health system.) Some of the barriers to setting up an integrated dated system are highlighted by Mendelson and Salinski (1997).

As a manager, you can help overcome barriers and facilitate the development and use of health information systems in your organization, community, or state and negotiate with other members of the system with regard to how and what types of data can be integrated. Choosing the right starting point is essential. Do not begin with a proposal to integrate health plan data that are proprietary. You will not get very far. Nor should you start with data that may be considered sensitive and confidential. Instead, you might start with aggregate data from health plans that give immunization rates for their enrolled population of two-year-old children. Alternatively, you could create a forum in which health plan data managers meet to develop a set of indicators to track tobacco use by minors. The skills that will make you successful in creating an integrated database will include negotiation, facilitation, networking, and knowledge of computer database systems.

Theme Two: Epidemiology

Epidemiology is one of the primary sciences that form the basis of public health. Public health epidemiology has traditionally focused on infectious disease. Now the discipline measures shifts in population demographics, health systems, and health outcomes. Collected data support health promotion, disease prevention, and program planning, implementation, and evaluation (Duncan 1998).

Epidemiology serves the community best when it functions in both the quantitative and qualitative domains. Quantitative data include counts and rates of occurrences of health status indicators. Qualitative data include information related to how people think, feel, or respond to occurrences of critical health problems. Using these data combined with monitoring and surveillance, public health leaders can measure whether the health status of the community is maintained or improved. Emerging health patterns can be identified early, making intervention more effective.

Once collected, the data must be analyzed to prioritize risks. You must ask these types of questions (Western Regional Center for the Application of Prevention Technologies 2000): What do the raw data tell us? How do the data compare with those from previous years? Is there a trend? How do the data compare with similar data at the regional, state, and national levels? What can we interpret from the data? Is there a relationship with another risk factor (*i.e.*, does increased incidence of communicable disease relate to decreased access to immunizations?)? Should this risk factor be prioritized?

Once data are collected and analyzed, they must be reported to those who will make decisions about how to use and prioritize the information they contain. The report should be in language that people outside the health professions will readily understand. Community members can relate to health status assessment reports when data are presented as health information. They are much closer to data that reflect their culture, norms, and values than they are to statistics about morbidity and mortality rates. As we begin to work more directly with communities, this skill in developing ways to portray information to audiences in ways that prompt action will be a key factor to success in building capacity within communities to take action on their health issues.

Finding a balance between quantitative and qualitative data can be challenging for epidemiologists. Your role as a manager is to assure that you have staff within your agency who can function in this capacity. In addition, you must assure staff have access to data and the means to analyze and report it. Without this type of information, you cannot fulfill one of your primary missions as a public health manager: to protect and promote the health of the community.

Management skills needed for this function include human resources management (*i.e.*, can you hire an epidemiologist who has experience with qualitative data?), developing a budget that contains funding for the tools of epidemiology (*e.g.*, computers, surveys, Internet capability, etc.), and the ability to communicate data to the community for decision making.

Theme Three: Implementing a Community Health Assessment

Everyone seems to be conducting community assessments these days. Community assessment is on the agenda of most health departments, some hospitals, and many health plans and has created a booming business for community development consultants. You must assure that your community is engaged in an assessment that will generate a plan for solving the top priority health problems identified. We have identified several health assessment models that can help you in this process. They all contain steps such as:

- Facilitate the creation of a community coalition that will commit to a community assessment process (minimum of a two-year commitment).

- Establish a staff work group who will support the community coalition.

- Access and/or create a community health profile of data indicators for use by the coalition.

- Identify the health problems important to the community and the assets the community brings to problem solving.

- Analyze each health problem and create effective interventions.

- Assure that responsibility for intervention is assigned to the most appropriate community partners.

- Measure the performance of each partner as it relates to success in mediating the health problem.

Whose responsibility is it to take action and facilitate this process? That responsibility may change once the process begins. However, if your community does not have such a plan for a regular community assessment, consider facilitating the start of the process. Once underway, it may be appropriate to relinquish the leadership to a community partner. The process will need to be staffed, and this may very well remain the responsibility of the health department. The skills required of you as a manager include facilitation, strategic planning, negotiating roles and responsibilities, and determining the appropriate role of the health department in setting priorities and creating interventions. You may find that your greatest challenge is sharing power with the community.

Learning Activity

The following activity addresses the assessment core function and includes indicators that can be used as measurable guidelines in evaluating the success of your community assessment.

Learning Activity #1: Indicators for Community Health Assessment

Using the information contained in appendices A and B, select four indicators you could use to measure the success of your community assessment. Remember that your indicators must be measurable within a specified time period. Caution: Health status improvement can take a long time, so think about indicators that measure intermediate health outcomes or measure the success of a process.

Describe each of your indicators, what data sources you would use in gathering information on your indicators, and whose performance the indicators measure.

Include a statement on how community involvement improves or changes outcomes.

References

Centers for Disease Control and Prevention (CDC). 1995. *Planned Approach to Community Health: Guide for the Local Coordinator.* Atlanta, Ga.: Centers for Disease Control and Prevention.

Duncan, K. 1998. *Community Health Information Systems, Lessons for the Future.* Chicago, Ill.: American College of Health Care Executives.

Mendelson, D., and E. Salinsky. 1997. Health information systems and the role of state government. *Health Affairs* 16(3): 106-119.

Missouri Department of Health. 1996. CHART: Community Health Assessment Resource Team. Retrieved on December 21, 2000, from the World Wide Web: http://www.health.state.mo.us/CHART/

National Association of County and City Health Officials (NACCHO). 2000. MAPP-Mobilizing for Action through Planning and Partnerships. Retrieved on December 29, 2000, from the World Wide Web: http://www.naccho.org/project49.htm

Washington State Department of Health. 1994. *Public Health Improvement Plan: A Blueprint for Action.* Olympia: Washington State Department of Health. (Available online at http://www.doh.wa.gov)

Western Regional Center for the Application of Prevention Technologies. 2000. *Building a Successful Prevention Program.* Retrieved on October 30, 2000, from the World Wide Web: http://www.open.org/~westcapt/naanalyz.htm

8

Managing the Policy Function

Objectives

- Describe the policy development core function.

- Identify the specific management skills involved in the policy development function.

- Articulate the specific legal authority for the public health director.

- Develop a policy options memo.

Essential Readings

Mahan, C. 1997. Surrendering control to the locals. *Journal of Public Health Management and Practice* 3(1): 27-33.

Washington State Department of Health. 1996. *Public Health Improvement Plan: A Blueprint for Action.* Olympia: Washington State Department of Health.

Wiesner, P. 1997. Public health leadership in DeKalb County. *Journal of Public Health Management and Practice* 3(1): 51-58.

First, let's do a quick review of policy development. The core function of policy development means that policy at the state and local levels is developed, implemented, and evaluated in a comprehensive manner. This includes making sure that administrative policies in organizations are congruent with state and local policy. Such policy development is based on both qualitative and quantitative scientific information and community values. The policy development function requires the ability to listen to residents who understand the strengths and weaknesses of those who live in the community. You must be able to prioritize work according to the needs of those in the community and build from the community's strengths. It is, after all, the people of any community who make the daily decisions that determine the health of the community. Residents who seek better health can organize themselves toward that end.

Public health policy is established through processes involving many individuals and organizations, including state and local boards of health, elected officials, community groups, public health professionals, health care providers, and citizens. This work is resource intensive. It requires dedicated staff and time for the community process to unfold. Public health jurisdictions must have the legal authority to make and implement policy decisions. Decision makers must evaluate information from health assessment activities and listen to the concerns expressed by community members. Furthermore, public health jurisdictions must be able to evaluate both planned and current policies. In order to do this, they must have the technical ability and resources to provide authorized decision makers with periodic information and data analysis regarding specific health issues. They must also have a system to facilitate community involvement and inform community members on a regular basis. State and local public health jurisdictions must have a similar framework for policy development activities, allowing for differences that result from their respective scope of responsibilities (Washington State Department of Health 1996).

We can think of policy development as a circular process. It starts with policy formation, the window of opportunity when the issue is on the community's agenda and the political circumstances allow solutions. The second phase is policy implementation, the development of plans, rules, regulations, and guidelines for implementing the strategies. The third phase is policy modification, evaluating progress toward policy goals and modifying the strategies when necessary (Lee et al.1999).

Two themes guide the study of managing policy development.

Theme One – Governance

The first theme revolves around your role with the public health governance body. In most cases, elected officials actually make policy; your role is to create options for them to consider and to influence, if possible, their decisions.

Theme Two – Legal Authority

The second theme has to do with assuring that your operating policies and legal authority give you the power to carry out your public health roles, including the authority to manage the policy development core function. Your role in policy development will be short lived if you do not have the legal authority for operating, and your governance board does not recognize or support the activities required to implement and enforce public health policy.

Theme One: Governance

Think of governance in two ways: (1) the power of an official body to direct, oversee, establish policy, and grant authority to government agencies including public health, and (2) the power of the community to directly influence the agencies that work for the benefit of the citizens. Public health agencies, therefore, respond to the official power of the legislative, executive, and judicial branches of government and to the legitimate power of the citizens.

As a leader in public health, you must organize your agency in such a way that it is responsive to the needs and desires of the population while following legal statutes and ordinances created by your official governance body. Being responsive to the community, as portrayed by Mahan (1997), can be a greater task than we might think! In this article, a state health officer views the local coalitions as his window to Florida's citizens and a reflection of the needs and desires of communities.

Mahan's narrative depicts the barriers that were overcome when control of maternal and child health decisions were turned over from state health office staff to local coalitions. The vision behind implementing coalitions was that more local control of health programs would help improve infant outcomes (Mahan 1997). However, the change represented a difficult leadership challenge. Responsibilities of the coalitions included assessing health care needs, establishing outcome objectives, developing health care service plans, organizing local provider networks, developing methods for allocating resources, and instituting a method to evaluate the effectiveness of services provided in the local jurisdiction. The efforts were extremely successful and generated numerous positive outcomes, including several infant mortality review projects, strong ties with the private sector, assurance of all pregnant women receiving prenatal care, and improved care for poor women (Mahan 1997).

Theme Two: Legal Authority

The major role of state agencies and local government is to carry out policy promulgated by elected officials. This policy will generally appear as law and the "rules" that guide implementation of the law. The laws and administrative codes grant power and authority to public health in your state. However, there may be a separation between this health policy authority and financial responsibility when public health does not receive supplemental resources to implement new mandates.

Your authority to act in your role as a public health leader depends on the ordinances and statutes that guide public health in your community or state. This authority is part of the governance structure of your public health system. What power and authority does your agency possess? How broad are those powers? Do rules developed to implement statutes allow for any self-determination or are they prescriptive? It is essential that the nurse leader become familiar with all relevant ordinances and statutes to guide policy development.

Learning Activities

Following are two learning activities to aid in your understanding of the core function of policy development. The activities specifically relate to governance and authority.

Learning Activity #1: Comparison of Strategies

Reflect on the Mahan and Wiesner articles listed in the Essential Readings. What similarities do you see between the strategies they employed as they respond to their governance issues?

Learning Activity #2: Policy Options Memo

To apply the themes of governance and authority in policy development, imagine that you are about to go before your local board of health with a recommendation that they consider a needle exchange program in your community. The board will ask you to help them understand what legal authority they and you have for such a program and will require you to bring them alternate options to a needle exchange program.

Use the options memo format on the following page to develop three policy options for your needle exchange program. One of your alternatives may be taking no action. It is important to have three viable options, one of which you will recommend. You would probably not include options that your department could not support.

Make sure you consider your target population and community stakeholders as well as data from your community assessment.

Policy Options Development

Developing an Action Options Memo

Your team has been instructed to develop an options paper for a needle exchange intervention. List three possible options and for each one address the issues identified below. Then select the best option and prepare the memo. Refer to the sample memo that follows.

Step 1 Assess Possible Action Options:

List three possible options.

For each, assess:

Technical feasibility

- Problem severity and urgency
- How well cause is understood
- How well technology is developed

Political feasibility

- Results of context mapping
- Clarity of legal mandate
- Buy-ins needed for implementation
- Impact on department

Budgetary implications

- Relative costs
- Potential availability of funds
- Impact on budgetary process

Step 2 Select Best Option:

Based on above analysis, compare the three options and select the most appropriate one.

Step 3 Prepare a brief memo:

- Identify key decision maker(s) to whom the memo should be addressed: who must approve before you can act?
- Briefly state nature of problem.
- Describe the <u>three</u> options.
- State your recommendation, why you selected it, and why you did not select the others.

Sample Policy Options Memo

November 26, 1994

To: Board of County Commissioners, sitting as the County Board of Health, and other interested parties.

From: Public Health Staff (Contact: Bill Jones)

This memo describes options linking the new Community Health and Safety Network to a local public agency to assure a stable funding source and recommends one of them. Action is scheduled for the Board meeting of December 27, 1994.

Background

The Youth Violence Prevention Act of 1994 mandates creation of a Community Health and Safety Network to serve as the vehicle for planning violence prevention and coordinating service provision in the county. The makeup, functions, and strategic role of the network have been the subject of continuing dialogue among interested parties for the past four months; the Department of Health has sponsored and chaired these meetings. Agreements have been reached that the Network will be governed by thirteen identified citizens and ten representatives from various local governments and agencies. The only major decision left before the Network is to choose a local public agency to serve as the Network's fiscal base. The statute requires that such an agency be specified at the inception of the Network.

Option 1

The City School District is a logical body to serve in this capacity and has offered to do so. The School District is included as a Network member and will have major responsibilities under any violence prevention plan that the Network develops. It has the staff and fiscal experience to handle Network financial needs.

Option 2

The City itself has made a strong argument to serve as the fiscal base for the Network. It, too, is a Network member and has the requisite staff and experience.

Option 3

The County Department of Health could also do the job and has several other specific statutory roles to play with respect to the Network and its functions.

Staff recommends Option 3 on the grounds of countywide responsibilities and account-ability, **but also suggests a proviso to be added**.

Option 1 is not recommended because there are three school districts involved in the Network and two others in the county, which chose not to be formally affiliated. Selecting the City School District might cause other districts to be less eager to participate, and would make the fiscal base accountable only to a relatively small number of voters

Option 2 is not recommended for the reasons stated above. Moreover, the principal reason that caused the City Council to ask for this role was the argument of the City Chief of Police to the effect that the business community needed assurance that its concerns about violent youth in the downtown area would be addressed by the Network. The Network is committed to doing so and should not allow its policies and priorities to be affected by its fiscal base in any event.

Option 3 is preferred because the county is the only public agency with countywide jurisdiction and accountability. The legislature is regularly addressing counties as regional units and has assigned the Department of Health a number of specific roles and responsibilities with respect to the Network. Serving as the fiscal base is quite consistent with these other special roles and will likely be accepted by the other participants.

We recommend adding a proviso to the Network articles of agreement to the effect that the Network can by majority vote request participating public agencies to contribute funds to a violence prevention account that the Department will maintain. Such contributions may never be needed because the state is currently giving high priority to violence-related efforts and both public and private funding are also relatively high, but the flexibility should be there in case the situation changes.

(Adapted from *Washington State Public Health Core Functions Training Coach's Manual* 1995, pages 106-7; permission granted by the Washington State Department of Health.)

References

Lee, P., A.E. Benjamin, and D. Barr. 1999. Health care policy in a changing world. In *Health and welfare for families in the 21st century*, edited by Wallace, H., G. Green, K. Jaros, L. Paine, and M. Story. Sudbury, Mass.: Jones and Bartlett Publisher.

Mahan, C. 1997. Surrendering control to the locals. *Journal of Public Health Management and Practice* 3(1): 27-33.

Washington State Department of Health. 1994. *Public Health Improvement Plan: A Blueprint for Action*. Olympia: Washington State Department of Health. (Available online at http://www.doh.wa.gov)

Washington State Department of Health. 1995. *Washington State Public Health Core Functions Training Coach's Manual*. Olympia: Washington State Department of Health.

9

Managing the Assurance Function

Objectives

■ Describe the assurance core function.

■ Identify specific management skills involved in the assurance function.

■ Develop a plan for determining how best to provide clinical care for the uninsured or underinsured within your community.

Essential Readings

Handler, A., and B. Turnock. 1997. Local health department effectiveness in addressing the core functions of public health: Essential ingredients. *Journal of Public Health Policy* 17(4): 460-483.

McLaughlin, D. 1996. A county health system director on Medicaid managed care. *Health Affairs* 15(3): 180-181.

U.S. Department of Health and Human Services. 2000. *Healthy People 2010, Conference Edition.* Washington, D.C.: U.S. Department of Health and Human Services.

Public Health Foundation. 2000. *Healthy People 2010 Toolkit: A Field Guide to Health Planning.* Washington, D.C.: Public Health Foundation.

University of Kansas. Community Tool Box. http://ctb.lsi.ukans.edu/ Accessed 10/30/00.

Assurance Function Components

The assurance function contains several complex components. In describing this multifaceted function, the Washington State Department of Health (1994) addresses three elements: administration, prevention, and access/quality.

To carry out its mission and form successful community partnerships, each public health jurisdiction must have a clear administrative structure that supports the core public health functions. Effective administration is a critical element of all efforts to improve and promote community health. Administration involves leadership, planning, and financial and organizational management. In addition, managers must clearly assign responsibilities, delegate authority, and develop operating policies and procedures.

The heart of public health is prevention of disease, injury, disability, and premature death.

- Primary prevention reduces susceptibility or exposure to health threats. Immunizations and family planning are examples of primary prevention.

- Secondary prevention most often detects and treats disease in early stages. A program to encourage the use of mammograms to detect breast cancer is an example of a secondary prevention activity.

- Tertiary prevention alleviates some of the effects of disease and injury through such means as habilitation and rehabilitation. An example would be a home visiting program for children with special needs.

Preventive services are provided to individuals in clinical settings, to families in home visits, and to groups of people in the community. The primary focus of public health prevention is to protect entire communities or populations from such threats as communicable diseases, unhealthy behaviors, epidemics, and environmental contaminants. Certain clinical personal health services are included because they benefit both the individual and the community. Immunizations, reproductive services, and communicable disease screening and treatment are examples of clinical personal health services that are of public health significance. The absence of these services can have wide ranging effects for the community as a whole.

Public health jurisdictions monitor and maintain the quality of public health services and participate in monitoring the quality of health and social services through credentialing and discipline of health professionals, licensing of facilities, and enforcement of standards and regulations. They also have a role to play in assuring that all residents have access to health services. Efforts to assure access and quality of care require partnerships among many affected

Assurance Function Subset	Components/ Themes
Administration	Structure that supports successful community partnerships and carries out its mission. Leadership, planning, and financial and organizational management.
Prevention	Primary, Secondary, and Tertiary. To protect individuals, families, and communities from infectious and chronic disease, injury, and unhealthy behaviors.
Access/Quality	Monitoring the quality of health services. Assuring that residents of communities have access to health care. Tracking of data.

parties, sharing of data, tracking of measurements, establishing programs, and implementing changes over time. They require ongoing efforts to obtain community and client perspectives on quality of care or services received (Washington State Department of Health 1994).

Three themes help describe the assurance function. The assurance function, with its administrative components, can be the key to successfully performing the assessment and policy responsibilities.

Theme One – Strategic Development and Action

Public health historically involves extensive population-based planning. Today's public health environment, however, requires action-oriented planning.

Theme Two – Strategic Management

Strategic management focuses on the development of a strategic outlook and planning for identified community issues.

Theme Three – Quality Improvement

An emerging role for public health is systems quality. We find ourselves more and more involved in assuring that the quality of the entire health system meets certain standards.

Theme One: Strategic Development and Action

Successful development of the organizational structures, financing, and workforce functions needed for public health demands that we be action- and strategy-oriented. Strategic development and action require us to be partners instead of the solo pioneers to which we are accustomed in public health. We must also be strategic in our choices of partners, approaches, and measures of success. We must bring together representatives of various community organizations to work jointly in solving our community's issues. The public health nurse leader must be able to build relationships among the different sectors, organizations, and constituents in the community. These alliances must be durable, structured, and issue oriented (Peterson and Alexander 1999). In other words, those plans must be implemented with associated measurable objectives, time lines, and assigned accountability.

Theme Two: Strategic Management

Leaders may think they have sole responsibility for determining the organization's strategies based on environmental cues. In fact, the leader who recognizes that staff can help read these cues and form solutions is much more likely to succeed. Nursing cannot expect to survive in an organization without all staff engaged in the process of recognizing and addressing the very subtle signals in the environment. Environmental cues occur regularly, and we may fail to detect them.

Nursing leaders must develop systems that assure flexibility and quick responses to problem areas. Recognizing that public health is not the only influence on the health of the community, nursing leaders must use a systems approach to address health concerns. Empowered staff operating in multiple community arenas may approach the health concern from different perspectives and achieve results not possible from a centralized bureaucracy. Building resiliency, instilling confidence, embracing risk taking, and assuming accountability are key strategies to a flexible and responsive organization.

In their article on local health department effectiveness, Handler and Turnock (1997) describe how some health departments address public health core functions. We must think about measuring our effectiveness in public health. Enlightened health plans are developing strategies to bring prevention activities to the communities they serve. Our ability to strategically align ourselves with those health plans will help assure that the most appropriate planning and implementation efforts are carried out and will also avoid duplication and/or competition.

Theme Three: Quality Improvement

Health plans, providers, and public health jurisdictions are accountable for the quality of their own programs. However, the overall responsibility for quality of the system that works to improve the health of all citizens often goes unassigned. Public health is a logical partner for this assignment because of our knowledge and commitment to population health. Many health departments are rethinking their role in primary care as evidenced by the number of health conferences devoted to the theme of managed care. The choices that must be made are provoking considerable anxiety in public health circles. McLaughlin (1996) writes about his viewpoint on managed care from the public health perspective. Many choices exist in terms of structuring health care and responding to the needs of the uninsured. Some choices are more positive for public health than others. All choices require a formal system for quality oversight.

The system of quality oversight includes the programs within your agency. Evaluation is indispensable for assessment, policy development, and assurance. Evaluation will tell you if the particular service, program, or system identified in policy was successful in achieving the outcomes for priority risks identified in the community assessment. A comprehensive evaluation also indicates what changes to strategies are needed to assure achievement of outcomes. If we look at evaluating the system of health care, we can document which elements of the system facilitate successful intervention for the community's risk factors. We will also be able to articulate the interrelationships among component parts that support achievement of policy objectives (Peterson and Alexander 1999).

Learning Activities

Two learning activities have been provided to ensure an understanding of the primary objectives of this chapter related to the core function of assurance.

Learning Activity #1: Access and Quality Capacity Standards

Read again pages 99 and 100 of the 1996 *Public Health Improvement Plan* (appendix C) and consider how you would carry out the access and quality capacity standards.

Learning Activity #2: Future Scenarios

Imagine facing two alternate future scenarios in which to test your management skills. You can join a regional health plan and begin doing a share of the uncompensated care in your community, or you can join forces with a community coalition that is planning to meet the safety net needs of the community through a network of providers in the medical care system.

The first scenario requires you to provide a percentage of the charity care stemming from a large population of uninsured individuals. If you choose this scenario, you must determine how you will support the charity care. If you develop a managed care business, how will you continue to support the core functions of public health?

If you choose scenario two, what role will you take in this planning process? How will you assure that access is managed appropriately by this network of providers? Choose one of these scenarios and sketch out your preferred outcome for the future. For the scenario you choose, determine what the budget implications will be for engaging in the required planning process.

References

Handler, A., and B. Turnock. 1997. Local health department effectiveness in addressing the core functions of public health: essential ingredients. *Journal of Public Health Policy* 17(4): 460-483.

McLaughlin, D. 1996. A county health system director on Medicaid managed care. *Health Affairs* 15(3): 180-181.

Peterson, D., and G. Alexander. 1999. Evaluation, performance monitoring, and health status surveillance. In *Health and welfare for families in the 21st century*, edited by Wallace, H., G. Green, K. Jaros, L. Paine, and M. Story. Sudbury, Mass.: Jones and Bartlett Publisher.

Washington State Department of Health. 1994. *Public Health Improvement Plan: A Blueprint for Action*. Olympia: Washington State Department of Health. (Available online at http://www.doh.wa.gov)

Afterword

Well, here we are at the end of the book.

Congratulations! You have completed what we hope has been a challenging and stimulating journey. It has been our intent to provide an opportunity for you to pause in your busy work world and reflect on your nursing practice and skills. We have provided information, learning activities, and resources for you to use to enhance your leadership of public health nurses, public health agencies, and communities. We encourage you to maintain your passion, to embrace change, and to harness its positive energy to innovate and create. It is our hope that you reach the end of this workbook feeling inspired and motivated to move forward with renewed vision about how to work effectively in your role as a nursing leader.

If we can be of any further help, please email us at bobbieb@u.washington.edu.

We want to wish you well as you go about changing the world.

Bobbie Berkowitz, PhD, RN, FAAN

Jan Dahl, MA, RN

Kay Guirl, MN, RN

Bonnie J. Kostelecky, MS, MPA, RN

Carol McNeil, BS, RN

Valda Upenieks, MN, RN

"Never doubt that a small group of thoughtful citizens can change the world. Indeed, it is the only thing that ever has." — Margaret Mead

Appendix A
Examples of System Performance Measures

Structure and Policies

Core Function	Standards of Performance (1994 Capacity Standards)	Indicators of Performance	Data Sources
Assessment	Policies, procedures, and legal authority guide the collection and use of data. (Capacity Standards 1, 2, 58, 61)	1. LHJ has identified procedures for information collection from data sources, the organization and analysis of information, and the transmittal of findings to data users. 2. LHJ has an established process to monitor and evaluate assessment activities to ensure their validity and accuracy.	• RCWs and WACs • BOH by-laws • BOH resolutions • LHJ and DOH policies, procedures, and standards
Policy Development	Processes to develop public health policy are defined, applied, and consistent with legal authority. (Capacity Standards 3, 15, 16, 21, 22, 29, 30, 37, 41, 48, 65-68, 76, 78)	3. LHJ has an identified process, which it uses, to develop policies that are presented to the Board of Health. 4. LHJ has an established system for the ongoing evaluation of priority public health issues.	• Policy and procedures manuals • BOH policies • Meeting minutes
Administration	Governance and management structures are in place that incorporate responsibilities and authorities of the Board of Health, Health Officer, and Administrator. (Capacity Standards 15, 16, 19, 20-22, 29, 30, 35, 37, 38, 41, 43)	5. Legally constituted Board of Health meets at least quarterly in an open forum that facilitates community participation in the meetings. 6. LHJ legal obligations such as compensation plans and contracts for services are approved by the Board of Health.	• RCWs • BOH meeting minutes • Resolution and motions adopted by BOH • Health Officer appointed pursuant to RCW 70.05
Prevention	Community health services are based on the jurisdiction's explicit authority, Board of Health authorization, and internal policies. (Capacity Standards 15, 16, 22, 29, 64, 66, 67, 71, 73)	7. LHJ prevention and protection programs are approved by the Health Officer, Administrator, and/or Board of Health. 8. LHJ prevention and protection programs are reviewed annually to assure they meet the intent of the statutes, regulations, and contractual requirements.	• Policy manuals • Local ordinances • BOH minutes • Contracts • Memoranda of understanding
Access and Quality	Policies, legal authority, and community action plans guide the assurance of access and quality of community health services. (Capacity Standards 74, 75)	9. LHJ has identified practices to assure community access to, and quality of, health services including prevention and protection.	• Plans addressing access and quality • Policy and procedures manuals • Job descriptions

Skills and Resources

Core Function	Standards of Performance (1994 Capacity Standards)	Indicators of Performance	Data Sources
Assessment	Assessment activities are performed by equipped and competent personnel. (Capacity Standards 1-7, 19, 23-25, 33, 34, 46, 50, 51, 58, 61, 65)	10. LHJ has access to people technically skilled in carrying out assessment activities. 11. LHJ acts to assure the availability of resources required to effectively perform assessment activities. 12. LHJ provides opportunities for continuing education and peer support to staff involved in assessment activities.	• Job qualifications • Personnel records • Continuing education records
Policy Development	Policy options are developed by equipped and competent personnel. (Capacity Standards 9, 18-20, 23-25, 41, 47, 81)	13. LHJ has access to people technically skilled in carrying out policy development activities. 14. LHJ acts to assure the availability of resources required to effectively perform policy development activities. 15. LHJ provides opportunities for continuing education and peer support to staff involved in policy development activities.	• Job qualifications • Personnel records • Continuing education records
Administration	Human resources, contracting, and procuring systems assure public health functions are performed by trained, equipped, and competent personnel in accord with contractual and legal obligations. (Capacity Standards 1-4, 7, 18-25, 32, 34-36, 40-45, 47, 58, 62)	16. LHJ has access to people technically skilled in carrying out administration activities. 17. LHJ acts to assure the availability of resources required to effectively perform administration activities. 18. LHJ provides opportunities for continuing education and peer support to staff involved in administration activities. 19. LHJ has a written description of the personnel and financial management systems.	• Written staff development plans • Continuing education records • Personnel records • Job descriptions • Written performance appraisal system
Prevention	Prevention programs are managed by staff who are skilled and knowledgeable in community health services. (Capacity Standards 3, 9, 45, 46, 49, 50, 53-60, 62, 65, 68, 69, 80)	20. LHJ has access to people technically skilled in carrying out prevention programs. 21. LHJ acts to assure the availability of resources required to effectively perform prevention programs. 22. LHJ provides opportunities for continuing education and peer support to staff involved in the core function of prevention.	• Personnel records • Job qualifications • Continuing education records
Access and Quality	LHJ uses skilled and knowledgeable staff to monitor and maintain the quality of community health services and to assure access and quality of care in the community. (Capacity Standards 74, 75)	23. LHJ has access to people technically skilled in carrying out the core function of access and quality. 24. LHJ acts to assure the availability of resources required to effectively perform the core function of access and quality. 25. LHJ provides opportunities for continuing education and peer support to staff involved in the core function of access and quality.	• Personnel records • Job qualifications • Continuing education records

Information and Communication

Core Function	Standards of Performance (1994 Capacity Standards)	Indicators of Performance	Data Sources
Assessment	Information systems enable the collection, use, and communication of data. (Capacity Standards 1-5, 19, 23-28, 33, 34, 46, 50, 51, 58, 61, 65)	26. LHJ systematically distributes public health data to the community providers, boards, and organizations serving the community.	• Policy and procedures manuals • Public relations documents, news releases, and presentation outlines
Policy Development	Public health policies are communicated within the public health community and to the community at large. (Capacity Standards 17, 18, 19, 28, 31, 34, 46, 50, 51, 86)	27. LHJ assures that the provider community received information on new, revises, and priority public health policies. 28. LHJ assures that Board of Health and staff members receive orientation to the role of LHJ in policy development.	• Written orientation and training procedures • Evidence of orientation • News releases and presentations
Administration	Information management enables oversight, planning, monitoring, and periodic evaluation of department policies and services. (Capacity Standards 1, 2, 4, 7, 19, 23-35, 27, 28, 31, 33, 34, 38, 40, 42, 46, 51, 58, 61)	29. LHJ management information systems track financial and service data. 30. Data from management information systems are analyzed, and information is developed for reporting to internal and external constituencies. 31. LHJs have the ability to communicate electronically with one another, the DOH, and the CDC.	• Management information system reports • State and local assessment data
Prevention	Prevention and protection services are consistent with community assessment and other data. (Capacity Standards 11, 33, 34, 51, 63, 72, 82, 84, 86)	32. LHJ uses data acquired through the information systems in the development of health policy and the evaluation of prevention services.	• Information systems reports • Project descriptions • Contracts • Project reports
Access and Quality	Local health jurisdiction and community providers collaborate on the collection and distribution of community health service data. (Capacity Standards 74, 76)	33. Local health providers are informed annually of progress to improve health priorities and strategies related to access and quality. 34. LHJ information system collects and distributes data on access to and quality of health services in the community.	• Services utilization data • Annual reports • Agreements with local providers • Resource directory

Community Involvement

Core Function	Standards of Performance (1994 Capacity Standards)	Indicators of Performance	Data Sources
Assessment	Community is involved in the assessment of its health. (Capacity Standards 3, 5, 6, 19, 23-28, 46, 50, 51)	35. LHJ provides opportunity to involve the community in the development of methods used to determine the extent and magnitude of local public health problems.	• Policy and procedures manuals • Community meeting minutes
Policy Development	Community health priorities are established through a community-wide process. (Capacity Standards, 6, 17, 25, 26, 27, 28, 48, 51, 61, 78)	36. LHJ assures that leaders in health care, government agencies, and the general public are involved in determining priority public health issues in the community.	• Budget • Community meeting minutes • Community assessment report
Administration	Financial practices support community priorities, and community involvement. (Capacity Standards 17, 23, 26, 28, 32, 39, 48, 61)	37. LHJ budget, reviewed and adopted by the Board of Health in a public process, reflects public health priorities.	• Meeting minutes • BOH resolutions
Prevention	Public health promotion and protection activities are appropriate for the community. (Capacity Standards 5, 25-28, 48, 61)	38. LHJ identifies and collaborates with constituent groups to address priority health promotion and protection needs in the community.	• Affiliation agreements • Contracts • Meeting minutes
Access and Quality	The combined efforts of the local health jurisdiction and the community are effective in assuring access to and quality of local health services. (Capacity Standard 76)	39. LHJ provides coordination, direction, and leadership within the community to improve the access to, and quality of, health services.	• Community mailing lists • Community meeting minutes • Program reports

Source: Reprinted with permission from the Washington State Department of Health, *Public Health Improvement Plan* (Washington State Department of Health, 1996), 82-85.

Guide to Acronyms:
BOH   Board of Health
CDC   Centers for Disease Control and Prevention
DOH   Department of Health
LHJ   Local Health Jurisdiction
RCW   Restricted Code of Washington
WAC   Washington Administrative Code

Appendix B
Examples of Health Status Indicators

Socio-Demographic Profile

1. Birth rate
2. Population (# and %) by 5-year age groupings for each sex
3. Population (# and %) by race/ethnicity
4. Household income by categories
5. Percent of population < 100% federal poverty level
6. Percent of population < 200% federal poverty level
7. Percent unemployed
8. Percent of persons over 25 years with high school diploma
9. Percent population change 1980-90 (or 95), overall and for age groups
10. Median income
11. Percent of persons at current address for at least 5 years
12. Percent of persons who moved into county within last 5 years
13. Percent retired
14. Divorce rate
15. High school drop out rate
16. Number of homeless shelter clients/rate per 100,000

General Health Indicators

1. Life expectancy
2. Overall death rate per 100,000
3. Top 5 causes of death – rate per 100,000 overall and by age/sex and ypll
4. Top 5 causes of hospitalization
5. Avoidable hospitalization per 100,000 population
6. Perceived health status
7. Percent of population without health insurance
8. Percent of population without usual source of primary care
9. Dental care indicator

Chronic Disease

Behavioral Risk Indicators

1. Percent of breast, cervical, and colorectal cancers diagnosed at a late stage
2. Percent of persons age 18+ who smoke
3. Percent of adolescents who smoke
4. Percent of women age 18-64 with pap smear in past three years
5. Percent of women age 50-64 with mammogram in past two years
6. Percent of population > 18 with blood pressure measured in past 2 years
7. Percent of population > 18 with cholesterol measured in past 5 years
8. Percent of persons reporting moderate, regular exercise

9. Percent of persons reporting obesity
10. Percent reporting they eat 5 fruit/vegetable servings a day

Disease/Outcome Indicators
1. Coronary heart disease deaths per 100,000
2. Stroke deaths – rate per 100,000 and ypll
3. All cancer deaths – rate per 100,000 and ypll
4. Lung cancer deaths – rate per 100,000 and ypll
5. Breast cancer deaths – rate per 100,000 and ypll
6. Colorectal cancer deaths – rate per 100,000 and ypll
7. Cervical cancer deaths – rate per 100,000 and ypll
8. Prostate cancer deaths – rate per 100,000 and ypll
9. COPD deaths – rate per 100,000 and ypll
10. Liver disease deaths – rate per 100,000 and ypll
11. Diabetes deaths – rate per 100,000 and ypll
12. Asthma hospitalizations – rate per 100,000 and ypll
13. All cancer cases – rate per 100,000 and ypll
14. Lung cancer cases – rate per 100,000 and ypll
15. Breast cancer cases – rate per 100,000 and ypll
16. Colorectal cancer cases – rate per 100,000 and ypll
17. Cervical cancer cases – rate per 100,000 and ypll
18. Prostate cancer cases – rate per 100,000 and ypll
19. Smoking-related deaths per 100,000

Maternal-Child Health

Behavioral Risk Indicators
1. Percent of mothers not receiving prenatal care during first trimester
2. Percent of mothers not receiving prenatal care by third trimester
3. Percent of mothers who smoked during their pregnancy
4. Percent of mothers who reported drinking during their pregnancy
5. Births by age categories (including category for teenagers)
6. Abortion rate
7. Percent of births delivered outside county
8. Percent of Medicaid children up to date with EPSDT or USPSTF screening
9. Income of mother

Disease/Outcome Indicators
1. Total infant mortality rate
2. Neonatal deaths (0-28 days)
3. Percent of live births < 2500 grams
4. Abortion rate
5. Percent of live births with congenital anomalies

Unintentional Injury and Poisoning

Behavioral Risk Indicators
1. Percent seat belt use in investigated collisions
2. Number of hazardous materials events (spills, drug labs)
3. Number of pesticide complaints
4. Number of pesticide investigations
5. Percent of drivers reporting seat belt use
6. Percent of bicyclists wearing helmets
7. Percent of water recreation facilities with identified critical item deficiency

Disease/Outcome Indicators

1. Unintentional injury deaths – rate per 100,000, age-specific rates, ypll
2. Unintentional injury hospitalizations – rate per 100,000
3. Firearm deaths – rate per 100,000, ypll
4. Motor vehicle deaths – rate per 100,000, age-specific rate, ypll
5. Residential fire deaths – rate per 100,000
6. Falling deaths – rate per 100,000
7. Falling hospitalizations – rate per 100,000
8. Drowning deaths – rate per 100,000 (natural water and recreational facilities) – coroner
9. Poisoning deaths – rate per 100,000
10. Poisoning hospitalizations – rate per 100,000
11. Unintentional CO poisoning hospitalizations – rate per 100,000
12. Number of children/adults identified with elevated blood lead levels
13. Occupational injury/illness claims per 100,000
14. Number of pesticide illnesses – rate per 100,000
15. Work-related injury deaths per 100,000
16. Number of reported traffic injury accidents

Infectious Disease

Behavioral Risk Indicators

1. Percent of 2 year olds with completed immunizations – by race, birth order
2. Risk indicator(s) for HIV/AIDS
3. Risk indicator(s) for STDs

Disease/Outcome Indicators

1. Incidence of chlamydia cases – number and rate per 100,000
2. Incidence of syphilis cases - number and rate per 100,000
3. Incidence of gonorrhea cases - number and rate per 100,000
4. Incidence of TB cases - number and rate per 100,000
5. Incidence of Hepatitis A and B cases - number and rate per 100,000
6. Incidence of pneumonia/influenza deaths - number and rate per 100,000
7. Incidence of pneumonia hospitalizations - number and rate per 100,000
8. Incidence of childhood vaccine-preventable illnesses - number and rate per 100,000 (HiB, diphtheria, tetanus, pertussis, measles, mumps, rubella, polio)
9. Incidence of Campylobacter - number and rate per 100,000
10. Incidence of E. coli - number and rate per 100,000
11. Incidence of Salmonella and rate per 100,000
12. Incidence of Shigella - number and rate per 100,000
13. Incidence of giardiasis - number and rate per 100,000
14. Rabies cases - number and rate per 100,000
15. Vector-borne disease - number and rate per 100,000
16. Zoonotic disease - number and rate per 100,000
17. Incidence of AIDS cases - number and rate per 100,000
18. Number of recreational - related waterborne disease outbreaks/cases per 100,000

Crime and Violence

Behavioral Risk Indicators

1. Miscellaneous indicators from Youth Risk Assessment Database
2. Miscellaneous indicators from Adolescent Health Behaviors Survey

Disease/Outcome Indicators

1. Homicide deaths – rate per 100,000, by age and race
2. Assault-related hospitalizations

3. Arrests/victims of violent crimes per 100,000, 10-17 year olds
4. Arrests/victims of violent crimes per 100,000, 18+ year olds
5. CPS reported cases of child abuse per 100,000
6. Arrests for domestic violence per 100,000
7. Additional indicators from Youth Risk Assessment Database
8. Number of calls for various crime/violence categories
9. Percent of crimes committed by county residents
10. Additional indicators for child/spouse abuse

Mental Health and Substance Abuse

Behavioral Risk Indicators
1. Miscellaneous indicators from Youth Risk Assessment Database
2. Miscellaneous indicators from Adolescent Health Behaviors Survey
3. Percent of persons reporting chronic drinking
4. Percent of persons reporting binge drinking
5. Percent of adolescents reporting alcohol use
6. Percent of adolescents reporting frequent alcohol use
7. Percent of adolescents reporting recent drug use
8. Percent of adolescents reporting frequent drug use
9. Additional mental health indicators from BRFS

Disease/Outcome Indicators
1. Suicide deaths – rate per 100,000
2. Alcohol-related deaths per 100,000
3. Mental health service utilization information from Regional Support Network
4. Number of mental health crisis line calls
5. Number of DWI arrests

Air Quality

Environmental Risk Indicators
1. Number of days of impaired air quality (exceeded EPA primary criteria standards)
2. Number of days wood burning in stoves is banned or restricted

Drinking Water Quality

Environmental Risk Indicators
1. Number and percent of households on Group A drinking water systems
2. Number and percent of households on Group B drinking water systems
3. Number and percent of households on individual drinking water systems
4. Number of complaints per year per 100,000 related to drinking water quality
5. Percent of households served by routinely tested water supply
6. Percent of households served by water supplies with optimal fluoride levels
7. Number and percent of systems not in compliance with Safe Drinking Water Act standards for failure to monitor bacteriological water quality
8. Number and percent of systems not in compliance with Safe Drinking Water Act standards for failure to monitor chemical water quality
9. Number and percent of systems not in compliance with bacteriological standards
10. Number and percent of systems not in compliance with chemical standards
11. Number and percent of Group A systems with vulnerable primary sources of drinking water

Disease/Outcome Indicators

1. Number of waterborne disease outbreaks
2. Number of waterborne disease cases/rate per 100,000

Food Quality

Note: Pending recommendations by E.H. Directors workgroup

Environmental Risk Indicators
1. Percent of inspections resulting in scores >35 critical violation points

Disease/Outcome Indicators
1. Number of food-borne outbreaks
2. Number of food-borne illnesses – rate per 100,000

Liquid Waste

Environmental Risk Indicators
1. Repair permits as percent of total systems
2. Percent of population served by sewage treatment plants
3. Percent of sewage treatment plants providing primary treatment only
4. Percent of homes surveyed for sewage system failures
   (including shellfish)/percent of failures

(Reprinted with permission from: Northwest Washington Epidemiology Partnership. 1997. *Regional Health Status Report for Island, San Juan and Skagit Counties.* Bellingham, WA.: Northwest Regional Council.)

Appendix C
Core Function Capacity Standards

These capacity standards differ slightly from those in the 1994 Public Health Improvement Plan. They were revised to improve clarity and specificity and to be consistent with current law. One standard has been added to "Administration" (no. 35), and two have been deleted in "Access and Quality."

Health Assessment

Health assessment means the regular collection, analysis, and sharing of information about health conditions, risks, and resources in a community. Assessment activities monitor, analyze, and evaluate community health status, risk indicators, and, when necessary, health emergencies. They identify trends in illness, injury, and death and the factors that can cause these events. They also identify environmental risk factors, community concerns, community health resources, and the use of health services. Assessment includes gathering statistical data as well as conducting epidemiologic and other investigations.

Assessment Capacity Standards

All public health jurisdictions, both state and local, must:

1. Have access to an integrated, centrally managed electronic network that provides access to federal, state, and local information systems.

2. Develop, operate, and assure the quality of data management systems that meet local needs to systematically collect, analyze, and monitor standardized baseline data.

3. Conduct and publicize epidemiologic, sociologic, economic, and other investigations that assess the health of the community and access to health care.

4. Link with local and statewide databases, such as vaccination registries, CDC INPHO system, vital records, and community hospital information systems.

Each local public health jurisdiction must:

5. Conduct a regular community health assessment using a standardized format such as the Assessment Protocol for Excellence in Public Health (APEX/PH).

6. Identify barriers in a community related to transportation, language, culture, education, information, and service delivery systems design that affect access to health services, especially for low income and other special populations.

7. Assure access to high-quality, cost-effective, timely environmental and clinical laboratory services that support outbreak investigations and meet routine diagnostic and surveillance needs.

The state must:

8. Develop community data standards as well as statewide standards for data use and dissemination. This should be a collaborative process with the Health Care Policy Board, health services purchasers, and the public health system. This includes standardized approaches to health status indicators, geographic information systems, population data, and biostatistical calculations.

9. Provide consultation and technical assistance to ensure a high standard of data analysis, dissemination, and risk communication.

10. Implement a fully integrated, secure statewide computer network that will include electronic mail, accessibility to documents and files, and the ability to access and amend basic data systems.

11. Evaluate and disseminate information regarding new health and information technologies in collaboration with organizations such as the Health Care Policy Board, CDC, State Board of Health, and health professions associations.

12. Survey the statewide availability of clinical and environmental laboratory services and help local health jurisdictions track this information.

13. Provide a public health laboratory that is closely integrated with the needs and requirements of state and local health jurisdictions.

14. Assess the supply and distribution of health care providers, facilities, and services.

Policy Development

A goal of the Public Health Improvement Plan is to assure that, at both state and local levels, policies are developed, implemented, and evaluated in a comprehensive manner that incorporates both qualitative and quantitative scientific information and community values.

The most effective public health jurisdictions are supported by the communities they serve. It is, after all, the people of any community who make the daily decisions that determine the health of the community. Residents who seek better health can organize themselves toward that end. Public health jurisdictions with the capacity to empower communities can assist in this effort.

This capacity requires the ability to listen to residents who understand the strengths and weaknesses of those who live in the community. It requires the ability to prioritize work according to the needs of those in the community and build from their strengths rather than from institutional strengths.

Public health policy is established through processes involving many individuals and organizations, including state and local boards of health, elected officials, community groups, public health professionals, health care providers, and citizens. Public health jurisdictions must have the legal authority to make and implement policy decisions. Decision makers must evaluate information from health assessment activities and listen to the concerns expressed by community members.

Public health jurisdictions must be able to evaluate both planned and current policies. To do this, they must have the technical ability and resources to provide authorized decision makers with periodic information and data analyses regarding specific health issues. They must also have a system to facilitate community involvement and inform community members on a regular basis. State and local public health jurisdictions must have a similar framework for policy development activities, allowing for differences that result from their respective scope of responsibilities.

Policy Development Capacity Standards

All public health jurisdictions, both state and local, must:

Authority

15. Develop explicit and formal statements of the public health jurisdiction's legal authority to develop, implement, and enforce public health policy.

Policy Analysis and Formulation

16. Enact policies and procedures within the existing legal scope of authority. There are two kinds of authority: authority granted to state and local boards of health to enact rules and authority to make decisions regarding those issues that do not require action by a board of health.

17. Involve the community in developing and analyzing policies related to the community's strategic plan and the jurisdiction's policy and planning activities.

18. Develop, analyze, and communicate alternative policies.

19. Provide accurate, timely, understandable information and data to policy makers, community leaders, and health care providers with emphasis on identifying threshold standards that have been exceeded. This includes technical support to decision makers to help them anticipate the effect of regulations, budget decisions, and policies on the community or the state as a whole.

20. Provide legal counsel to review policy decisions.

21. Promote state and local legislation and regulation aimed at reducing public health risk factors and promoting healthy behaviors. Evaluate current legislation and regulation to determine if it supports these goals.

Policy Implementation

22. Translate enacted policies into operating program procedures including:

    - Clarify or establish the legal basis and authority that are required to proceed with implementation.

    - Define and estimate the costs of personnel, equipment, and facilities associated with procedures that have been developed.

23. Estimate the costs and effects of proposed policies, secure resources to support these policies, and inform affected parties and the community.

Policy Evaluation

24. Identify policy outcomes, develop outcome measures, evaluate them on a regular basis, and communicate the findings.

25. Evaluate the program efforts:

    - To assure that they address community needs and problems.

    - To assess the relative efficacy, costs, and benefits between specific prevention programs as well as between prevention programs and medical treatment.

Community Collaboration and Mobilization

26. Mobilize the community and in particular health care providers in a systematic and periodic process to set community priorities, develop policies, and formulate strategies to address key public health problems based on the community assessment.

27. Collaborate with community members and health care providers to inform the public about the current health status of the community, using formats appropriate to the needs of various individuals or organizations.

28. Provide information and data, as requested and appropriate and in keeping with confidentiality requirements, to interested community groups for health-related activities.

Administration

To carry out its mission and form successful community partnerships, each jurisdiction must have a clear administrative structure that supports the core public health functions. Effective administration is a critical element of all efforts to improve and promote community health. It involves a number of important features, including leadership, planning, and financial and organizational management. All of the capacity standards assume that an effective administrative structure is in place. This is especially true of Policy Development, which includes key standards concerning community leadership and planning. Responsibilities related to the internal workings of the public health jurisdiction require the same leadership and management skills: agency and division directors must clearly assign responsibilities, delegate authority, and develop operating policies and procedures.

Administration Capacity Standards

All public health jurisdictions, both state and local, must:

Agency Management

29. Secure policy board authorization for operation of programs.

30. Periodically assess the role of other units of government within the agency's jurisdiction and their respective authority to implement public health policies to improve and promote community health.

31. Regularly collect and analyze information describing agency and program administration, funding, activities, workloads, client characteristics, and service costs.

32. Develop a long-range strategic plan and time-limited, measurable agency and program objectives.

33. Assure the collection, analysis, and use of information that is needed to evaluate the outcome of program activities on risk and protective factors and health status.

34. Maintain a management information system and electronic communication capacity that allows the analysis of administrative demographic, epidemiologic, and service utilization data to provide information for planning, administration, and evaluation.

35. Participate in agreements with other jurisdictions, as appropriate, to manage costs.

36. Secure and maintain qualified administrative and health officer leadership.

Financial Management

37. Designate a person who is responsible to oversee all financial responsibilities of the health jurisdiction.

38. Develop and implement a long-term financial plan (i.e., extends beyond the operating budget cycle) that is consistent with the strategic plan identified in Standard 32.

39. Develop and implement budgets that reflect jurisdictional priorities and programs, address health problems, and assure that expenditures follow the budget and financial plan.

40. Involve professional and community groups in development, presentation, and justification of the budget.

41. Develop and manage contracts to provide public health services to or for community organizations, private nonprofit corporations, and health care organizations.

42. Assure that the policy board and staff understand their legal accountability and liability as well as their general responsibility to the public for wise financial management.

Personnel Management

43. Have a comprehensive system of personnel management that complies with appropriate federal, state, and local regulations, including documenting relationships with other units or departments of government that carry out personnel functions of the public health jurisdiction.

44. Have an established working relationship and labor agreement between the health jurisdiction policy board and, where applicable, each labor union representing staff.

45. Maintain a salary administration plan authorized by the policy board and designed to attract and retain competent staff.

46. Develop and implement a staffing plan that includes recruitment and retention strategies and professional development opportunities.

Prevention

The heart of public health is prevention of disease, injury, disability, and premature death. Prevention includes:

- Primary prevention, which reduces susceptibility or exposure to health threats. Immunizations are an example of primary prevention.

- Secondary prevention, which most often detects and treats disease in early stages. A program to encourage the use of mammograms to detect breast cancer is an example of a secondary prevention activity.

- Tertiary prevention, which alleviates some of the effects of disease and injury through such means as habilitation and rehabilitation.

Prevention services are provided both one-on-one in clinical settings and to groups of people in the community. The primary focus of public health prevention is to protect entire communities or populations from such threats as communicable diseases, epidemics, and environmental contaminants.

Certain personal clinical health services are included in the standards because they benefit both the individual and the community. Immunizations, reproductive services, and communicable disease screening and treatment are examples of services that are of public health significance. The absence of these services can have wide-ranging effects for the community as a whole.

Two main components of primary prevention are health promotion and health protection.

Health Promotion

Health promotion includes health education and the fostering of healthy living conditions and lifestyles. Health promotion activities may be directed toward individuals, families, groups, or entire communities. They help people identify health needs, obtain information and resources, and mobilize to achieve change. They foster an environment in which the beliefs, attitudes, and skills represented by individual behavior and the community norms are conducive to good individual and community health.

Health promotion includes communicating surveillance and epidemiologic data to public health officials, other health providers, industries, and the community as a whole. It includes working with communities on an on-going basis to communicate relevant information, helping their mobilization efforts, and providing technical assistance and consultation.

Health Promotion Capacity Standards

All public health jurisdictions, both state and local, must:

47. Assure that the public is informed of the health status of the community and relevant health issues and that education is provided regarding positive health behavior.

48. Assure the development and provision of culturally, linguistically, and age-appropriate health promotion programs for community health priorities.

49. Collaborate with public and private agencies, health care purchasers, and providers to develop strategies to address public health risk factors.

50. Assure provision of services that enhance healthy family relationships and child growth and development.

51. Provide education and information to the general public about communicable and non-communicable diseases of public health importance.

Each local public health jurisdiction must:

52. Maintain an information and referral system concerning available health facilities, resources, and services.

The state must:

53. Provide health promotion models to address public health risk factors.

54. Assure that health promotion programs addressing health risk factors and positive healthy behaviors are implemented statewide consistent with locally identified health priorities by providing technical assistance and program support.

55. Assure that continuing education programs are available that address disease and injury prevention to meet the specific needs of caregivers, health and facilities professionals, and other public and private partners.

56. Promote the use of K-12 school health education curricula.

Health Protection

Health protection refers to those population-based services and programs that control and reduce the exposure of the population to environmental or personal hazards, conditions, or factors that may cause disease, disability, injury, or death. Health protection also includes programs that assure public health services are available on a 24-hour basis to respond to public health emergencies and to coordinate responses of local, state, and federal organizations.

Health protection includes immunization, communicable disease surveillance, outbreak investigations, water purification, sewage treatment, control of toxic wastes, inspection of restaurant food service, and numerous other activities that protect people against injuries and occupational or environmental hazards.

Health protection activities occur throughout the community in homes, schools, recreation, and work sites. Because of this variability and the shared responsibility for safety, health protection activities require collaboration with many community partners.

Health Protection Capacity Standards

All public health jurisdictions, both state and local, must:

57. Perform monitoring, inspection, intervention, and enforcement activities that eliminate or reduce the exposure of citizens to communicable disease and environmental hazards in both routine and emergency situations.

    - Develop protection programs, in accordance with federal guidelines and scientifically identified risk factors, that address priority health risk factors.

    - Assure that communicable disease contact investigation and follow-up is performed in a timely and appropriate manner, in adherence to guidelines of the federal Centers for Disease Control and Prevention.

    - Assure that persons identified to have communicable diseases are given information about treatment protocols, provided with prompt and effective treatment when available, and advised about appropriate behavioral changes to reduce the risk of disease transmission.

58. Assure that individuals, especially children, are immunized according to recommended public health schedules.

59. Assure the surveillance, diagnosis, and treatment of communicable diseases of public health significance.

60. Assure the provision of public health services that affect the community and high-risk populations, including:

    - Consultation and education services to day care centers and schools;

    - Intervention with high-risk families to provide standardized screening and assessment, education, counseling, and referral (e.g., NCAST, Minnesota Parenting Inventory, Region X Child Health Standards);

    - Community education on risk and harm reduction behavior;

    - Outreach to individuals not accessing care.

61. Assure provision of reproductive health services in the community.

62. Collaborate with communities in developing local and statewide emergency response plans, including mobilizing resources to control or prevent illness, injury, or death.

63. Provide on-going public health staff training in emergency response plans, including participation in practice exercises on a routine basis.

64. Provide 24-hour telephone access to respond to public health emergencies.

65. Conduct inspections, monitoring activities, and compliance strategies consistent with state and local board of health rules and regulations.

Each local public health jurisdiction must:

66. Identify and control potential and actual hazards to public health, such as maintaining a safe water system, ensuring safe food handling practices in restaurants, and managing toxic spills.

The state must:

67. Coordinate with federal rule-making agencies and the Congress to assure that they take

into account the effects of federal rules and statutes on the health risks, protection needs, and resources of Washington State.

68. Develop, in cooperation with local health jurisdictions and health care providers, statewide regulations and policies that guide the public health activities of direct service providers, the local public health jurisdictions, and state agencies.

69. Carry out direct regulatory responsibilities in environmental health programs, including those imposed by federal mandate, that are not addressed by local jurisdictions.

70. Assist communities in developing emergency medical and trauma care services to provide immediate access to life saving interventions for illness or injury.

71. Support and assist local agencies' crisis response efforts:

    • Support local health agencies in the provision of laboratory services, food and water inspection, radiological assessment, and disease identification and testing during emergencies.

    • Help coordinate the transfer of needed personnel, resources and equipment to emergency sites.

72. Designate the Department of Health as the lead agency, in the Washington State Comprehensive Emergency Management Plan, for coordinating all public health activities during emergencies.

73. Provide public information support to the Office of the Governor and to other state or federal emergency management agencies during emergency and disaster recovery operations.

74. Help coordinate and incorporate local emergency response plans into the Washington State Comprehensive Emergency Management Plan.

Access and Quality

Public health jurisdictions monitor and maintain the quality of public health services and participate in monitoring the quality of health and social services through credentialing and discipline of health professionals, licensing of facilities, and enforcement of standards and regulations. They also have a role to play in assuring that all residents have access to health services.

Efforts to assure access and quality of care require partnerships among many affected parties, sharing of data, and tracking of measurements, programs, and changes over time. They require on-going efforts to obtain community and client perspectives on quality of care or services received.

Access and Quality Capacity Standards

Each local public health jurisdiction must:

75. Assure that prevention and intervention efforts (including treatment) for communicable diseases and other public health conditions, are being appropriately implemented.

76. Assure the competence of food handlers, solid and hazardous waste generators, on-site sewage system designers, and other individuals whose activities fall within the public health authority of the local health jurisdiction.

77. Collaborate with health care providers and other community service agencies to reduce barriers to accessing health care and to assure that individuals and families are linked with health services.

The state must:

78. Assure access to personal primary and preventive health services. This includes:

    - Providing policy, financial, and technical support to help improve access;

    - Supporting community efforts to address unmet health needs;

    - Collaborate with health care training programs, professional organizations, health care providers, and community leaders to assure an adequate supply and distribution of high-quality provider services.

79. Establish criteria to assess the competency of health professionals as well as design, implement, and evaluate credentialing and certification methods for health professionals, facilities, and providers of other public services.

80. Assure that local health jurisdictions, contractors (including state-funded public health programs), health care sites, and providers comply with appropriate regulations and standards and meet contractual obligations.

81. Promote best practices through the use of professionally adopted standards of care.

82. Assure that health care and public health providers have access to and use on-going training.

83. Conduct quality assurance activities and operate state-mandated regulatory programs necessary to ensure that all laboratories produce high-quality outcomes. Work with agencies to correct deficiencies and provide appropriate training programs.

84. Improve the analytical performance of clinical and environmental laboratories through training, consultation, technology transfer, and regulation.

85. Promote the on-going use of utilization review, treatment outcome research, and performance-based program evaluations to achieve continuous quality improvement in public health and medical care services.

86. Evaluate health system workforce trends and determine effect on access to health care.

87. Designate the Department of Health as the primary advocate, along with other state agencies and public entities whose activities are intended to improve health status, to develop policies and programs that are consistent with population-based approaches to community health status improvement.

(Reprinted with permission from: the Washington State Department of Health, *Public Health Improvement Plan*. Washington State Department of Health, 1996.)

Appendix D
Annotated Bibliography

Changing Health Care Environment and Impact on Public Health

1. Beauchamp, D. 1997. Public health, privatization, and market populism: A time for reflection. *Quality Management in Health Care* 5(2): 73-79.

    The author critically discusses the concept of "market populism," the popular political, economic, and social ideology that places the free-market model of competition as the driving force for change in health care reform. The author asserts that this market populism ideology is the "most serious threat to public health in many decades." The author also considers the crucial implications for public health, pointing out that local and state health departments are those most seriously threatened by the forces of market populism. Suggestions are offered for public health professionals acting within their roles as advocates and protectors of the health of the public. These suggestions include steps taken to avert the dangerous consequences posed by increasing privatization, which further weakens public health infrastructure. The author remarks that increased assumption of a population-level focus within managed care may well serve to protect the public health of enrolled populations—yet adequate safeguards to protect the health of total populations are not assured.

2. Halverson, P.K., A.D. Kaluzny, G.P. Mays, and T.B. Richards. 1997. Privatizing health services: Alternative models and emerging issues for public health and quality management. *Quality Management in Health Care* 5(2): 1-18.

    This article critically examines the implications of movement of publicly funded health services into the private sector. An in-depth discussion of public health issues raised by mass privatization is provided. Some critical questions raised by the authors include:

    - How will privatization impact the public sector's capacity to serve the uninsured/underinsured and hard-to-reach populations?

    - How will privatization of personal health services erode funding sources for public health agencies, thereby threatening their ability to perform critical public health activities such as community assessment, policy development, communicable disease tracing, environmental health, and special population-focused planning and programs?

    - Are private sector providers able or willing to assume responsibility for the health care needs of clients traditionally served in the public sector?

    - How willing are private providers to afford health services and programs that may be unprofitable to them, particularly in the short-term?

    - Will privatization result in a decline in accessibility and availability of health services traditionally provided in the public sector?

- How will privatization affect the role of public health agencies—movement to oversight and enforcement?

The authors also describe factors within the health care marketplace and public/private health care organizations that give rise to the movement of privatization. In addition to addressing these implications and concerns, the authors discuss the strengths and weaknesses of a range of models through which privatization and quality improvement may occur and outline the instrumental role of public health agencies in creating and sustaining privatization initiatives.

Core Functions and Public Health Role Performance

3. Halverson, E.S., P.K. Kaluzny, C.A. Miller, B.J. Fried, S.E. Schenck, and T.B. Richards. 1996. Performing public health functions: The perceived contributions of public health and other community agencies. *Journal of Health and Human Services Administration* 18(3): 288-303.

This article discusses the results of an on-going study by a group of investigators of public health departments at the University of North Carolina. The investigative team developed a set of indicators to estimate levels of performance of core public health practices within local health departments. Information for this evaluation was collected from health department directors to estimate the contribution of non-public health agencies to overall performance of public health. Non-public health or "outside agencies" were identified as other state and local governmental agencies, physicians, clinics, and hospitals.

The findings of this investigation conclude that "outside agencies" provide approximately one-quarter of local public health activity. It is interesting to note that "adequacy of overall public health performance is significantly related to the extent of participation by outside agencies" (300). The core function in which the most significant level of activity has been recognized is in the policy development core function, the second being the assessment function. The authors summarize the study findings by remarking that only a small portion of public health practice is demonstrated by primary care providers. Furthermore, it was concluded that within the context of the "changing patterns of health care," public health activities will need to be more thoroughly incorporated into managed care practices, or local public health agencies will need to continue in their current role of assuring public health protection. The most salient point is made in the conclusion, when the authors state, "Local public health departments can maximize the impact by better understanding the nature of working relationships with multi-institutional arrangements, encouraging greater levels of collaboration and integration, and acting as catalysts for increased support of public health activities" (303).

4. Turnock, B., and A. Handler. 1997. From measuring to improving public health practice. *Annual Reviews of Public Health* 18: 261-282.

Turnock and Handler discuss the past and present challenges of measuring public health practice. The article highlights that prior to the Institute of Medicine's 1988 report, data concerning public health practice had emphasized measurement of immediate results of local public health services. The authors of this article argue that a shift in approach to measuring public health practice must occur, and the focus must be on performance related to public health's core functions. The authors further state that a standardization of this approach in the form of a comprehensive national surveillance system for public health practice is in demand. This surveillance system will need to both measure and examine the relationships among inputs, core function-related processes, outputs, and outcomes.

Partnerships and Collaboration

5. Courtney, R., E. Ballard, S. Fauver, M. Gariota, and L. Holland. 1996. The partnership model: Working with individuals, families, and communities toward a new vision of health. *Public Health Nursing* 13(3): 177-186.

   The authors discuss in detail the concept of partnership in public health. The traditional relationship of "professional-to-client" is contrasted with the concept of partnership. Several challenges faced by public health professionals related to accepting and engaging in this role transformation are addressed. An example of the partnership process is provided through a community-based project in an urban Hispanic community.

6. Kang, R. 1995. Building community capacity for health promotion: A challenge for public health nurses. *Public Health Nursing* 12(5): 312-318.

   This author discusses the role of the public health nurse within the core functions. Emphasis is placed on community capacity, noting that nurses must rise to this challenge. This can be accomplished through facilitating community participation, enhancing community health services, and coordinating public policy. Additional themes addressed in this article include:

   - Public health nurses must assume a key role in implementing the core functions of public health.

   - The concepts of health, community, participation, and partnership are clearly defined and used as the framework to define the focus for capacity-building efforts.

   - The role of public health nurses is addressed as building community capacity separately and within each core function.

7. Kotchian, S. 1997. Perspectives on the place of environmental health and protection in public health and public health agencies. *Annual Reviews of Public Health* 18: 245-259.

   This article describes the separation of environmental health from the field of public health and the current relationship of these two distinct entities. The article outlines the history of environmental health, its involvement within the field of public health, its eventual separation from other public health programs with resulting benefits and consequences, and possible outcomes concerning future environmental health and protection activities. A central theme in this article is that environmental health and public health professionals must work together to insure sustainability of human health.

8. Polivka, B., C. Kennedy, and R. Chaudry. 1997. Collaboration between local public health and community mental health agencies. *Research in Nursing and Health* 20: 153-160.

   This article describes a study concerning a proposed model of interagency collaboration. The conceptualization of this model contains five major constructs: environmental health, situational factors, task characteristics, interagency processes, and outcomes. Interagency collaboration was explored between public health agencies and community mental health agencies using this model. The study revealed that public health and mental health agencies (independent yet complementary) are not well linked and have few interagency referrals, tense relationships, and minimal goal congruence.

   Several key factors related to the process of interagency collaboration are relevant to public health nurse leaders attempting to collaborate across agencies:

   - Staff from different agencies should be able to identify each other; awareness of goals and responsibilities of these agencies and individuals, with which one is expected to collaborate, is essential for success.

- Official contracts between agencies that explicitly state which organization will assume which responsibilities when planning or implementing a program are important. (This is directly relevant to public health departments attempting a program with other direct care services.)

- The agreement must be a collaborative effort, more than just a contract—a shared process. Satisfaction with interagency collaboration was found to be directly affected by the extent of interagency processes.

- Assisting staff of one's own agency to recognize the value of interagency collaboration and more specifically the value of the roles that individuals from other agencies fill is an important element of the process.

9. Wasserman, M. 1997. Building a statewide coalition for tobacco control, 1993-present. *Journal of Public Health Management and Practice* 3(4): 8-13.

This article provides an example of a public health leader who created an action-oriented statewide coalition aimed at tobacco control. This leader describes the steps involved in building this coalition and the successes that resulted. The collaborative effort set forth positive outcomes in the areas of legislative advocacy and regulation. Residents through the workplace, as a result of smoking bans, felt the impact statewide, and laws were implemented restricting minors' access to tobacco. This article represents an example of a public health leader "leading" a group of diverse individuals and a variety of constituencies toward established goals. An important lesson learned was that the implementation phase was crucial for coalition building and involved a "building consensus" of group goals and plan for action.

Policy Development

10. Gebbie, K. 1997. Building a constituency for public health. *Journal of Public Health Management and Practice* 3(1): 4-11.

This case study recounts the experiences of a former public health director for the Health Division of Oregon Department of Human Resources. The author stresses the importance of building a broad constituency for public health as an essential strategy for public health leaders who require public and agency-wide support to achieve population level health improvements. The author relates several challenging situations during the period he served as public health director and describes the assortment of skills needed to commit to a long-term vision and implementation of actions. The range of strategies and skills required for successful constituency building included strategic planning and communications, long-term thinking and planning, community development activities, coalition building, media relations savvy, and more.

The article offers rich guidance for public health nursing staff and leaders in developing their roles as policy advocates. Multiple lessons may be drawn from this case study and applied to organizational policy development and change, community relations, and legislative policy activities.

Public Health and Managed Care Systems

11. Keener, S.R., J.W. Baker, and G.P. Mays. 1997. Providing public health services through an integrated delivery system. *Quality Management in Health Care* 5(2): 27-34.

This article describes a case example of a county government's decision to privatize the public health department under a state-owned, integrated health system conglomerate serving twelve counties across two states. The county's goals in privatizing the delivery of public health services included: (1) curb the annual growth of services in the community; (2) maintain the provision of high-quality public health services in the community by transferring the responsibility of performing the majority of public health functions from the health department to the county health system; (3) eliminate duplication of services; (4) create economies of scale; (5) realize inefficiencies through cost-shifting; and (6) exercise "organizational agility."

The author further elaborates on three built-in mechanisms for quality management, referred to as "strategies," which consisted of the following: (1) county's governance and advisory structure; (2) implementation of extensive internal evaluation and monitoring system (maintained jointly by a major university health service research center); and (3) statewide public health report card system.

12. Leong, D., and E. Lewis. 1996. *Health Systems Oversight: A Job For Public Health In The Managed Care Era—Skills Needed By The Public Health Work Force.* Washington, D.C.: Health Resources and Services Administration.

This report discusses the future role of public health departments as leaders in public oversight of managed care organizations. According to the authors, the transformation of the health care system into managed care, driven by the drive to reduce health care costs, has created new roles for public health nurses. These roles focus on the need to assure quality service provision, facilitate collaboration for systems change, and create policy changes necessary to continue to fulfill the central mission of public health.

A model for "health systems oversight" by public health is described that involves three central components: (1) systems protection—regulator; (2) systems assessment—surveyor; and (3) systems development—developer. The tenets of this model resemble the public health core functions of assessment, policy development, and assurance, all framed within a systems change approach. The authors outline and discuss an extensive list of skills required for the public health workforce that they developed from literature review and conversations with state and local health department staff.

Public Health Nursing Leadership

13. Miesner, T., J. Alexander, A. Blaha, P. Clarke, C. Cover, G. Felton, S. Fuller, J. Herman, M. Rodes, and H. Sharp. 1997. National Delphi study to determine competencies for nursing leadership in public health. *Image: Journal of Nursing Scholarship* 29(1): 47-51.

This article describes a study conducted to determine competencies needed by nurse leaders in public health programs. The findings resulted in fifty-seven competencies clustered into four groupings: political competencies, business acumen, program leadership, and management capabilities. The authors conclude that the findings provide data for curriculum development and evaluation of programs to prepare nurse leaders for roles in public health delivery systems. Although these findings provide a framework for the education of public health nurse leaders, the authors state that the competencies described are extremely relevant to practicing leaders.

14. Stevens, R. 1995. A study of public nursing directors in state health departments. *Public Health Nursing* 12(6): 432-435.

This author speaks to the challenges facing public health nursing to provide leadership in the changing public health environment. This article describes the result of a study aimed at identifying the current structure of public health nursing in a state health department in the United States. The results highlighted that neither policy input development nor creating a budget is an expectation of public health nurse leaders. In addition, emphasis is placed on the demand of public health nurse leaders to position themselves to influence policy. The study concludes that no uniform description exists of what states expect of their state nurse directors, even though these individuals lead the largest portion of the public health workforce.

15. Wallinder, J. 1997. Supporting one another: The definition of public health nursing, awards, and the impromptu. *Public Health Nursing* 14(2): 77-80.

This editorial presents the recently updated 1996 statement of the Public Health Nursing section of the American Public Health Association on the role and definition of public health nursing practice. A brief definition defines public health nursing as "the practice promoting and protecting the health populations using knowledge of nursing, social, and public health sciences" (78). The statement describes the steps and principles that guide the public health nursing process, discusses the many roles that public health nurses assume, and lists examples of nursing activities that are performed in collaboration with a host of community players. The intent of this article is to help public health nurses develop a clearer sense of the future roles and responsibilities of public health nursing within an increasingly interconnected environment of health care and public health systems.

Quality Improvement

16. Hatzell, T.A., E.S. Williams, P.K. Halverson, and A.D. Kaluzny. 1996. Improvement strategies for local health departments. *Quality Management in Health Care* 4(3): 79-86.

This article promotes the employment of quality improvement strategies within the local health departments as beneficial means for improving organizational effectiveness, efficiency, and adaptability within a rapidly changing health care environment. The many challenges confronting local public health departments resulting from changes within the current health care system are discussed in some depth and include: (1) shrinking public health resource bases, particularly for primary health care; (2) increased market competition for the position of personal care service provider to populations previously cared for by health departments; and (3) concentrated emergence of public health threats strongly associated with social causes. A host of internal factors associated with health departments' organizational structures, funding mechanisms, culture, and administration are also considered by the authors to contribute negatively to overall performance and reputation.

According to the authors, quality improvement strategies must be employed to enhance efficiency and demonstrate benefits to the community. Core public health functions provide the framework to guide strategic planning for quality improvement efforts. Additional crucial dimensions of quality improvement require the following: (1) staff to be thoroughly trained and supported in their efforts; (2) adoption of a strong service orientation to all service provision, which is community guided and responsive; (3) improvements in information collection, documentation, and management; and (4) empowerment and support of staff to creatively and collaboratively problem solve.

17. Kaluzny, A.D., C.P. McLaughlin, and K.I. Simpson. 1992. Applying total quality management concepts to public health organizations. *Public Health Reports* 107(3): 257-264.

The authors describe the total quality management approach to organizational improvement. Further, they explicitly state that total quality management is a powerful transformative tool widely used for "managerial innovation" that creates positive changes within public health agencies. The approach emphasizes accountability at the process, teamwork, and empowerment of staff.